Prostate Cancer and the Man You Love

Prostate Cancer and the Man You Love

Supporting and Caring for Your Loved One

2nd Edition

Anne Katz, PhD, RN, FAAN

ROWMAN & LITTLEFIELD
Lanham • Boulder • New York • London

Published by Rowman & Littlefield
An imprint of The Rowman & Littlefield Publishing Group, Inc.
4501 Forbes Boulevard, Suite 200, Lanham, Maryland 20706
www.rowman.com

86-90 Paul Street, London EC2A 4NE

British Library Cataloguing in Publication Information Available

Library of Congress Cataloging-in-Publication Data Available

ISBN: 978-1-5381-6390-0 (cloth)
ISBN: 978-1-5381-6391-7 (epub)

For my one and only

Contents

Chapter One

Introduction

This chapter explains the basics of prostate cancer to prepare you for reading the rest of this book. It contains an accessible description of the development of prostate cancer, screening for the disease, and how the pathology results and imaging studies guide the stage and grade of the cancer that in turn dictates treatment options. The various treatment options are described as well as the impact of each treatment's side effects on the couple.

Prostate cancer is a very common cancer in men, second only to skin cancer. It is most often diagnosed in men over the age of fifty years, and men of African American and Caribbean African ancestry are at high risk of developing this cancer. There may be a link to a family history of prostate cancer but most men will develop this cancer, regardless of family history. There are some identified genetic risk factors; men who carry the BRCA1 and BRCA2 genes as well as those with Lynch syndrome are at higher risk of developing prostate cancer. Other risk factors with less evidence include being exposed to Agent Orange or chemical agents associated with firefighting. Being an older man remains the greatest risk factor, and this cannot be modified or prevented!

WHAT AND WHERE IS THE PROSTATE GLAND?

The prostate gland lies below the bladder and surrounds the top part of the urethra (the tube that drains urine from the bladder). The prostate produces a fluid (seminal fluid) that nourishes sperm; during orgasm the prostate contracts and propels the semen out of the penis through the urethra. The prostate gland is about the size of a walnut and often increases in size as the man ages. This causes the man to need to urinate more frequently as well as incomplete emptying of the bladder. Prostate cancer, however, is not commonly accompanied by any symptoms at all, and men are often shocked when they are diagnosed because they had no warning that something was wrong.

PSA SCREENING

The PSA (prostate-specific antigen) test is a blood test that is used to screen for the presence of the PSA protein that can be a warning sign of prostate cancer. Both the prostate and prostate cancer cells produce this protein. The PSA test is plagued by low accuracy with both false positive and false negative results. A false positive result will cause anxiety in the patient as he waits for another test, a biopsy, that will show if he has prostate cancer or not. A false negative result may mean that a diagnosis is missed. There are cutoffs based on age for the PSA: for a man in his forties, the PSA should be between 0 and 2.5 ng/ml; for a man in his fifties, it can be as high as 3.5 ng/ml; for a man in his sixties, the normal range is between 0 and 4.5 ng/ml; and for a man in his seventies, it can range between 0 and 6.5 ng/ml. If the amount of the protein in the blood is raised, the man should have a biopsy of the prostate, a diagnostic test, that shows whether there is cancer in the prostate gland.

BIOPSY OF THE PROSTATE

A biopsy is required to diagnose prostate cancer. In this procedure, twelve or more samples of tissue are taken from the prostate. The biopsy has traditionally been performed using ultrasound to ensure that the samples are taken from specific areas in the prostate. During the biopsy, a probe is inserted into the rectum and tissue samples are taken from the prostate using long needles. Local anesthetic is injected into the area surrounding the prostate to minimize pain, but men often report that the procedure is still painful. The pain may be worse if the man is anxious (Chestnut 2020); this likely affects most men who have this procedure. A biopsy is not without risk. Because the biopsy needles go through the wall of the rectum, infections are possible. This is why men are prescribed antibiotics for the procedure; but even with this, a small percentage of men may develop an infection and may need to be hospitalized for treatment.

The ultrasound does not clearly show the location of cancer cells, so, more recently, using multiparametric magnetic resonance (MRI) imaging to guide the biopsy allows for more accurate targeting of any lesions in the prostate (Goldberg et al. 2020). This improves the identification of higher-grade prostate cancer and provides more information to guide treatment. An MRI does not use radiation but, instead, uses radio waves to produce a series of images that are then studied by the radiologist, and a report is sent to the provider who requested the MRI. The radiologist uses the Prostate Imaging Reporting and Data System (PI-RADS) to score the MRI. The PI-RAD score goes from 1 (most likely not cancer) to 5 (very suspicious for cancer).

THE GLEASON SCORE

The Gleason score is a measure of the aggressiveness of prostate cancer found from the biopsy. A pathologist looks at the tissues from the biopsy and assigns a grade between 3 and 5 to the area of the sample that has the most cancer cells. Cancer cells look different from normal cells, and the degree of abnormality is described as patterns 3, 4 or 5. Then, the pathologist looks at the area that has the second highest volume of cancer cells and, once again, assigns a number between 3 and 5 to those cells. The two numbers are then added (for example, $3 + 4 = 7$) and this number is known as the Gleason score. Gleason scores (the sum of the two numbers) range from 6/10 to 10/10. This number reflects the aggressiveness of the cancer, with 10/10 being the worst.

A newer system of grading has been developed (Kryvenko and Epstein 2016) and is approved by both the International Society of

Table 1.1.

Group 1	Gleason score $3 + 3 = 6$	Low-risk prostate cancer
Group 2	Gleason score $3 + 4 = 7$	Favorable, intermediate-risk prostate cancer
Group 3	Gleason score $4 + 3 = 7$	Unfavorable, intermediate-risk prostate cancer
Group 4	Gleason score 8	High-risk prostate cancer
Group 5	Gleason score 9 and 10	Very high-risk prostate cancer

Urological Pathology and the World Health Organization (Chen et al. 2018). The grading comprises five groups representing Gleason scores between 6 and 10 and is suggested to be clearer to both physicians and men with prostate cancer.

The biopsy report usually contains what percentage of cancer cells is contained in each sample. Consideration of how many samples contain cancer (e.g., 3/12) and how much volume there is in each sample (e.g., 10 percent or 1 mm) is used to help the physician recommend a certain treatment.

The use of biomarkers is an area of interest for screening, diagnosis, and treatment decision-making in prostate cancer. There are many tests to identify biomarkers available as well as even more in development. Most use either urine, blood, or tissue samples. However, there are still questions about the validity of these tests—how they compare to each other as well as their costs and, thus, affordability. Two of these tests, Prolaris and Oncotype DX, provide information about which men with positive biopsies need to be treated and which can be monitored (Kohaar, Petrovics, and Srivastava 2019).

It is important to remember that the existence of a test does not guarantee it will provide useful information.

TREATMENT DECISION-MAKING

In order to make a decision about treatment, the man needs to be fully informed about his cancer and the risks and benefits of the various treatments (Gnanapragasam 2020). This knowledge can help the man adopt positive coping mechanisms and reduce uncertainty about his illness (Guan et al. 2020). Shared treatment decision-making is regarded as important for men with prostate cancer. This involves the physician, the man with prostate cancer, and his family or other caregivers, as appropriate. The process involves providing the man and his supporters with enough information about his cancer to make a decision based on his values and preferences (Orom et al. 2016). It should not be assumed that the man has the knowledge to understand the intricacies of the various treatment options—their risks and their benefits. Providing his family/ caregiver(s) with the same information allows them to understand the challenges facing the man with prostate cancer as he makes a treatment decision. With this knowledge—about both treatment options and the challenges being faced—family/caregiver(s) may be better equipped to effectively modify their behavior in order to influence the man's decision in productive ways. It can be very difficult for a man to decide about treatment, and many men do not know that they have a choice. Some may prefer to be told by the doctor what treatment to have and do not want to share in the treatment decision-making process.

The role of health care providers other than physicians in the treatment decision-making process is also important (Thera et al. 2018). Nurse navigators have been shown to increase knowledge, provide reassurance, and decrease indecision. They are described as empathetic and trustworthy, and they provide information to the man that is individualized. Primary care providers, by virtue of the continuity of care they provide—which enhances their awareness of the person's values and preferences for treatment as well as their quality of life and relationships with family members—also play a potentially important role in the decision-making process (Merriel and Gnanapragasam 2019).

Urologists report that they encourage family members to be present at appointments and also encourage him to seek a second opinion. However, some physicians may find it difficult to talk with men and their family members because they know that receiving a cancer diagnosis is life-changing and carries an emotional burden (Adsul et al. 2017). Family members may influence the man's treatment decision. Thus, the information they have about the stage and grade of the cancer, how aggressive it is, and the treatment choices available is important. Lack of knowledge may lead to family pressuring the man to have a treatment that may not be effective for him. Family members want what is best for the man but also for themselves; longevity for the man has benefits for family members who love and care for him, and this may influence their actions and advice. Because men with prostate cancer have multiple treatment choices, they often seek the opinion of friends. Men are often heavily influenced by their friends, especially those who have also had prostate cancer, and it has been shown that consulting nonprofessionals creates more indecision and greater difficulty choosing a treatment (Reamer et al. 2017).

There are different factors that influence the treatment decisions of men with prostate cancer. One of these is the accuracy of their knowledge about their cancer. Many men do not understand the side effects of the various treatments (Daum et al. 2017) or their potential impact on quality of life (Shevach, Weiner, and Morgans 2019). Other factors influencing the man's decisions about treatment include the cost of treatment, how long the treatment takes, and recovery time (Gordon et al. 2019). It may be uncomfortable for health care providers to talk about the costs of treatment, and it is not clear that people with cancer take the costs into consideration when making a treatment decision (Imber et al. 2020), but the direct and indirect financial costs of treatment (called financial toxicity) are increasingly being realized as a serious consequence of treatment for cancer.

The role of the partner is very important in the process of deciding about treatment. In heterosexual couples, women play three roles: the first is that of counselor (offering advice); the second is that of confidant (providing emotional support); and, finally, that of coordinator (arranging appointments) (Bergner et al. 2018). If the man's partner is lacking information or support, this can affect the couple's relationship and may increase illness uncertainty for the man (Varner et al. 2019). Same-sex couples may see a different role for the partner, but there is no research to base this on.

There are a number of effective treatments for prostate cancer that you will read about in the following chapters. And because the treatment of prostate cancer results in side effects that have an impact on quality of life, men are encouraged to make their own choices about treatment. This can be frustrating for loved ones who are afraid that any delay could result in poor outcomes for the man. But studies have shown that a delay of several months, or even years, for men with low-risk prostate cancer is not harmful (van den Bergh et al. 2013), and for men with high-risk prostate cancer, delaying treatment is safe for up to six months (Xia et al. 2020). You and/or your family members may not agree with this!

Often, the man accepts the recommendation of the physician who is involved in his care, usually a urologist. However, he may not have enough information about the side effects of the recommended treatment (Hoffman et al. 2018), and this may lead to regret, later, when he experiences bladder leakage or sexual problems. Being actively involved in the decision-making process has been shown to result in satisfaction with treatment and quality of life after treatment (van Stam et al. 2018).

ACTIVE SURVEILLANCE

Active surveillance refers to conservative management of low-risk prostate cancer that is usually slow growing and does not pose a significant risk to the life of the man (Klotz 2017). This monitoring of the cancer delays or defers surgery or radiation, preserving his quality of life. Patients should be carefully selected for this protocol after test results and a comprehensive discussion about the benefits and risks (Merriel et al. 2021). Test results should be discussed with the man and his partner/spouse to assess his willingness to agree to delaying or deferring treatment.

Regular monitoring of the PSA and digital rectal examinations are recommended while the man is on active surveillance. If the PSA rises or a subsequent biopsy shows progression, the man then must decide whether he wants definitive treatment (surgery or radiation).

There have been studies looking at how many men stop active surveillance and have definitive treatment (surgery or radiation). In a large Canadian study, 36 percent of men on active surveillance had surgery or radiation therapy because of a rise in PSA and higher grade of prostate cancer on subsequent biopsy (Matta et al. 2020). Active surveillance may not be suitable for African American men due to a higher incidence of aggressive disease in these men (Shen, Pettaway, and Chen 2020). It is important that men follow the recommendations for follow-up tests, including biopsies (Detsky et al. 2020).

The research about how men on active surveillance cope with regular monitoring suggests that some men see a decrease in anxiety as time passes (Marzouk et al. 2018). While it is normal to experience anxiety initially (Ruane-McAteer et al. 2017), this may not last beyond the first few months after diagnosis. Men will often cope with anxiety by seeking clarity from their health care provider. They may do this by asking for information about their cancer and details about the protocol for active surveillance and triggers for treatment. Clarity and understanding lead to a sense of control that may help to minimize uncertainty. Trust in the health care team is also important as well as support from family (Wade et al. 2020).

It is important to understand that active surveillance is not "doing nothing" (Mallapareddi et al. 2017); it is a strategy to maintain quality of life and avoid the side effects of surgery or radiation for as long as possible.

RADICAL PROSTATECTOMY

A radical prostatectomy involves removing the entire prostate gland and the seminal vesicles. The surgery can be performed as an open procedure, where an incision is made from the below the umbilicus (belly button) to the pubic area. In the early 1990s, laparoscopic surgery became more common, in which instruments are inserted via small (keyhole) incisions in the abdomen to remove the prostate. More recently, robotic-assisted surgery has become popular, with 70 percent of radical prostatectomies in the United States using this technique (Sebesta and Anderson 2017); a robot is used to guide the instruments that are inserted into the body.

SIDE EFFECTS OF SURGERY

One of the most common side effects of the surgery is incontinence or bladder leakage. Most men will need to wear a pad or adult diaper for some time after removal of the urinary catheter; the Continence Product Advisor website (https://www.continenceproductadvisor.org/prostatecancer) provides guidance on how to deal with this. It may be useful for the man to keep a voiding diary that may show triggers for the incontinence. Lifestyle changes may help to reduce leakage; these include avoiding alcohol and other bladder irritants, restricting fluid intake, and not smoking (Radadia et al. 2018). Pelvic floor physiotherapy has been shown to be effective for men with prostate cancer experiencing incontinence after surgery, especially if started *before* the surgery (Milios, Ackland, and Green 2019; Manley et al. 2016). Modifications to the basic instructions for the exercises (known as "Kegel exercises" to many) include the use of resistance bands (Pan et al. 2019). Guidance by a pelvic floor physiotherapist is especially important because merely reading instructions is not effective for doing the exercises correctly (Wu et al. 2019).

Erectile difficulties are common after surgery, but there are other sexual side effects that are not usually discussed. These include shortening of the penis (El-Khatib et al. 2021) and loss of skin sensation on the penis, loss of orgasms or orgasm intensity, sometimes to the point of pain (Frey et al. 2014; Nolsøe et al. 2021). Some men lose some urine when they are aroused (Bach et al. 2019) and this is often very distressing (Salter, Bach, Katz, et al. 2020). Loss of urine with orgasm is also possible, and this may be bothersome to the man's partner as well (Jimbo et al. 2020; Salter, Bach, Miranda, et al. 2020). About 10 percent of men will notice curvature of the erect penis after surgery.

Men often assume that their erections will be the same as before surgery, but this occurs in only a small number of men (Nelson et al. 2013). Even if the man does see the return of erections, the often unspoken side effects, as described above, may negatively impact his overall sexual function and satisfaction (Fode et al. 2017). Despite the hope that robotic surgery would cause fewer erectile problems for men, it is suggested that outcomes have not improved to any great degree (Capogrosso and Salonia 2019). This highlights the importance of comprehensive pretreatment education of the man so that he has realistic expectations of erectile recovery after surgery.

Despite early promise in small studies, penile rehabilitation has not resulted in much improvement either. This involves taking a small dose of one of the medications for erectile dysfunction every night for two or more years. Many men do not continue with the nightly medication due to costs and lack of improvement (Klotz et al. 2005). Men may want to return to the same level of function that they had before the surgery, but only about a third of men achieve this (Terrier et al. 2018). Some men find it difficult to be satisfied with their sex life in the absence of spontaneous sexual intercourse; the planning and timing required when using medication or devices detracts from what they think of as "normal sex."

A staged approach to treating erectile problems is common. The first intervention are oral medications such as Viagra, Cialis, Stendra, and Levitra. These medications do not cause an erection but rather prevent blood from leaving the penis after penile stimulation. All of these medications have side effects including headache, indigestion, and facial flushing. If these don't help, a more invasive approach is taken with the penile pump, urethral tablets (MUSE), or penile self-injection. The option of last resort is a penile implant, a surgical procedure in which a mechanical device is inserted into the penis (Pillay et al. 2017).

Buying medications for erectile problems on the internet is not something that anyone should do. There is no guarantee that the pills purchased from an unknown source (despite fancy websites, often stating that the medication is coming from Canada) contains the active ingredient in Viagra or other medications. It may contain an unsafe higher dose or fillers that are dangerous to health.

RADIATION THERAPY

There have been many advances over the years in the methods of administration of radiation therapy; intensity modulated radiation therapy (IMRT) and stereotactic body radiation (SBRT) are types of external beam radiation. Brachytherapy, a form of internal radiation, refers to the insertion of tiny metal seeds directly into the prostate; each seed emits radiation that kills the cells. The radiation sources for external beam radiation include the linear accelerator, the Cyberknife robotic system, and the Gamma knife (Podder, Fredman, and Ellis 2018). Because of these different methods of providing radiation to the prostate, the decision about what method to use is left to the radiation oncologist who is the expert; men should be informed about the rationale for the specific kind of radiation treatment. For example, men with high-risk prostate cancer may be offered what is called a "brachytherapy boost" in addition to the course of external beam radiation (Greenberger, Zaorsky, and Den 2020). Some men may also need to have medication to suppress their testosterone in addition to the radiation treatment (Chen 2019).

Men and their partners have the need for accurate and timely information about the timing of the radiation and side effects of treatment (Gordon, Dickinson, and Offredy 2019). The major side effects of radiation are increased frequency of urination and bowel movement changes. When comparing the side effects of surgery and radiation at three years after treatment, men who had either treatment had similar quality of life. Sexual function and incontinence are worse for men who had surgery rather than radiation (Barocas et al. 2017). Men who have external beam radiation therapy have the same urinary and bowel function as those men who were on active surveillance in the years after treatment (Hoffman et al. 2020). One concern for men who have radiation therapy is the association of radiation with the development of a secondary cancer. There may be an increase in the risk for rectal cancer ten years after radiation therapy (Zhu et al. 2018). Men who need to urinate frequently during the night before treatment may experience worse urinary symptoms after radiation therapy. Men who smoke, use medication to treat heart disease and/or high blood pressure, or who have diabetes are more likely to experience urinary problems after radiation therapy (Rancati et al. 2017).

Sexual side effects may also occur. Erectile problems are found to occur in almost two thirds of men after external beam radiation (Budaus et al. 2012); brachytherapy appears to have less of an impact on erectile function with more than three quarters of men reporting that they are able to have an erection five years after treatment (Bazinet et al. 2020).

Urinary, bowel, and sexual side effects are known to cause distress for men (Orom et al. 2018) and this is often not disclosed to health care providers or family members due to the stoicism expected of men in Western society. It is suggested that counseling men about sexual side effects of radiation before treatment commences and encouraging the use of medication for erectile dysfunction, as well as exercise and a healthy diet, and also couples counseling can be helpful for men who choose radiation therapy (Nguyen et al. 2021). Increasing age, erectile function before treatment, and the dose of radiation have an impact on the return of erections after radiation therapy.

Proton therapy has been suggested as causing fewer side effects than traditional radiation therapy (Verma, Simone, and Mishra 2018) but the evidence supporting this is limited and studies suggest that the side effects are the same (Matta et al. 2019). Relatively few centers have the ability to provide this due to the high costs of construction and the costs to patients that are about twice as much as traditional radiation therapy (Royce and Efstathiou 2019) and this treatment may not be covered by insurance (Kamran, Light, and Efstathiou 2019). Other treatments include HIFU (high intensity focused ultrasound) and cryotherapy. Careful selection of men who are eligible for these treatments means that one cannot assume that these are effective treatments for all men with prostate cancer (Jung et al. 2018; Tourinho-Barbosa et al. 2020).

CANCER RECURRENCE

After both radiation and surgery, a rising PSA suggests that a recurrence of the cancer has occurred (Fakhrejahani, Madan, and Dahut 2017). A biochemical recurrence means that the recurrence has been detected based on a blood test rather than physical evidence. It is important for the treating physician to exclude the presence of metastatic disease (cancer that has spread beyond the prostate, often to the bones) in planning further treatment. Unfortunately, ultrasound, or CT scans, are usually not sensitive enough to detect the location of the cancer cells causing the recurrence. PET scans may be helpful for this (Lindenberg et al. 2017). More recently, PSMA PET-CT scans that use a contrast medium have been found to be useful in assessing whether there has been spread outside the prostate, but they may not be available outside of academic hospitals (Rans et al. 2020).

People often look for a cause of the cancer coming back and thinking about something that has changed in their behavior. There are some things that can help to prevent a recurrence and you may be key in encouraging him to do the following:

1. Maintaining a healthy body weight is likely the most important thing the man can do, for both his heart as well as preventing death from prostate cancer. Vigorous physical activity (activities that cause sweating and increased heart rate and breathing) is also associated with a lower risk of dying from prostate cancer.
2. In terms of diet, limiting the amount of red meat consumed, especially processed meat, is a good choice. Eating cooked tomatoes, especially if they are cooked in oil to increase absorption, may be of benefit. There is a caution to this: many of the studies about diet and prostate cancer look at diet in *reducing* the risk of getting pros-

tate cancer—we do not know as much about diet and recurrence of prostate cancer.

3. One factor that is associated with recurrence of prostate cancer is tobacco use. Men who smoke ten cigarettes a day for twenty years have a 75 percent chance of their cancer coming back (Khan, Thakkar, and Drake 2019). The longer a man smokes, even if he stops at some point, is associated with recurrence of cancer. And, of course, a history of smoking is also associated with heart and lung disease, including lung cancer.

ANDROGEN DEPRIVATION THERAPY

Testosterone, the male hormone or androgen, is necessary for prostate cancer cells to grow. If the cancer recurs, most men will be prescribed medication to deprive the cancer of its fuel. Sometimes called "hormone therapy," a more accurate name for the treatment is "androgen deprivation therapy"; by stopping the body's production of testosterone, prostate cancer cells are deprived of the fuel for growth (Crawford et al. 2019). These medications are given in the form of injections, but there are some newer forms of this treatment in pill form. Before these medications were developed, surgical removal of the testicles (orchiectomy), where the majority of testosterone is made in men, was the method used to reduce testosterone levels. While this procedure costs less than years of medication, it has a psychological impact on men (another word for the surgery is "castration") and is not reversible.

Anti-androgen treatment in the form of pills is usually given before starting the injections that stop testosterone production in the body. These medications are also called androgen-receptor blockers or nonsteroidal anti-androgens. They block the testosterone receptors in the testicles where most of the body's testosterone is produced. This is necessary because if the level of testosterone in the body drops suddenly after the injection, the body will try to produce more to restore the level of the hormone in the body; this is called a "testosterone flare." This is not good when the man has prostate cancer as it may cause the cancer cells to increase.

Once the anti-androgens block the receptors for testosterone in the body, the man is given the testosterone blocking medication. These medications are known as LHRH-agonists (these go by the trade names Lupron, Elligard, Zoldaex, Trelstar, or Camcevi) or LHRH-antagonists (their trade names are Firmagon and Orgovyx). See the American Cancer Society website for more details (https://www.cancer.org/cancer/prostate-cancer/treating/hormone-therapy.html).

There is a long list of side effects for these medications but men may not experience all of them. Breast tenderness that occurs with the androgen receptor blockers usually decreases when the man starts the injections of testosterone-reducing medication. Some men find that wearing a tight T-shirt or undershirt can help to bind the breast tissue and decrease pain with movement. In more severe cases, radiation therapy to the affected area(s) can be helpful, although there is a risk that the radiation can damage the heart (Tunio et al. 2012).

One of the most common side effects of androgen deprivation therapy is hot flashes, affecting up to three quarters of men (Fankhauser et al. 2020). Described as a feeling of heat that occurs suddenly and is accompanied by sweating and flushing, they are distressing to men and often continue long after treatment is over. They also result in interrupted sleep (Gonzalez et al. 2018), which may have an impact on the sleep of a partner sharing the same bed. Poor sleep quality also has an effect on daily energy, causing an increase in fatigue (Dickinson 2021).

There are limited interventions for the treatment of hot flashes (Qan'ir et al. 2019). Medications such as antidepressants may be helpful for some men; acupuncture may be more helpful for others. Some men find that spicy foods and indoor heating trigger their hot flashes (Magee and Singal 2020), so avoiding these may be helpful. Wearing layers can also help men cope with the feeling of being hot; deep breathing at the onset of a hot flash has been shown to be helpful (Wibowo et al. 2019). Using a fan in the bedroom can also help as well as choosing bed linen with a low thread count, which allows for better air circulation.

Alterations in mood (irritability or anxiety) is another side effect of androgen deprivation therapy (Cherrier and Higano 2020). Men may report poor appetite, worry, and intrusive thoughts, and while these may seem to suggest that he is depressed, the man may deny this. There is an increased risk of depression for men on androgen deprivation therapy (Nead et al. 2017), and there is also an increased risk of suicide, especially in older men who live alone (Klaassen et al. 2018). Depression magnifies the impact of other side effects such as loss of masculinity that result from the sexual side effects of the medication (Siebert, Lapping-Carr, and Morgans 2020).

A decline in cognitive functioning has been seen in men on this treatment, specifically in the areas of verbal memory (causing word loss), attention, and executive function (making decisions) (Mundell et al. 2017). There has been some concern that the medication may be associated with the development of Alzheimer's disease and other forms of dementia (Nead, Sinha, and Nguyen 2017) but the association is not clear cut (Kluger, Roy, and Chao 2020). Men and their partners/ spouses need to be told that there may be a risk of dementia, and they need regular assessment of cognitive function while on androgen deprivation therapy.

Weight gain, especially in the abdominal area, is a common side effect of the lack of testosterone. This can cause problems with body image, something that men may be reluctant to talk about (Gentili et al. 2019). The larger issue of feminization of the male body (growth of breast tissue, loss of upper body muscle mass, loss of body hair, and softening of the skin) is also distressing to men, who may be reluctant to report this. Men may be concerned about how they are judged by others and may avoid exercising in public. They may feel the need to change their style of clothing, avoiding knit fabrics or anything that might cling to the body, and/or they may need to buy new clothes because of their weight gain.

These changes are more than physical; weight gain and loss of lean muscle mass are known factors involved in the metabolic syndrome that is associated with cardiovascular (heart) health (Edmunds et al. 2020). The risk of cardiovascular disease is increased in men on androgen deprivation therapy, especially those who are elderly (Gupta et al. 2018) and those with preexisting cardiovascular disease (Melloni and Roe 2020).

Reducing the risks of weight gain is focused mostly in the area of exercise; regular exercise has been shown to prevent further weight gain as well as to increase physical fitness and muscle strength (Cormie and Zopf 2020). It is suggested that merely encouraging men to engage in physical exercise is not enough; referral to an exercise specialist who can create an individualized exercise plan and monitor the man's progress is more likely to be successful. An exercise regimen should include aerobic activities, resistance training, and weight-bearing exercise (Owen et al. 2017). Eating a balanced diet, with a focus on fruits and vegetables and a low fat intake, in addition to exercise may help to prevent further weight gain and potentially lead to weight loss (Wilson et al. 2021).

Loss of bone mineral density and the development of osteoporosis is another side effect of androgen deprivation therapy (Joseph, Lam, and Patel 2019). It is recommended that men take calcium and vitamin D supplements to prevent bone density loss. Exercise alone has not been shown to be effective in preventing bone mineral density loss but has many other general health benefits (Bressi et al. 2021; Geerkens, Pouwels, and Beerlage 2020).

CLINICAL TRIALS

Men may be offered participation in a clinical trial at some point during their cancer treatment; the trial may be investigating a new drug or procedure. The new treatment will be tested against an existing one, so while the man is part of an "experiment," he will still be receiving an effective treatment, whether or not he receives the experimental medication. It is not ethical to test a cancer drug against a placebo (or sugar pill) because that would deny the person any treatment.

Before the study or clinical trial can begin, the researchers need to get approval from an institutional review board, which is often part of a university or may be a private company that reviews research. Members of the review board are usually doctors, researchers, and patient advocates, and they are independent of the researchers doing the trial. The review board ensures that the research is ethical and conducted according to the rules and laws that have been made to protect research participants. An investigational new drug (IND) application also needs to be sent to the Food and Drug Administration (FDA) for approval. The FDA reviews details of the proposed study, including whether the trial team has the skills and knowledge needed to conduct the study as well as to see if the participants will be exposed to risks that can be harmful and avoided.

Clinical trials are divided into three types: phase 1, 2, and 3. In a phase 1 trial, participants (usually healthy volunteers) are given the new drug to see if it is safe and at which dose it can be given. Phase 1 trials often happen in the hospital or a special clinical trial unit where participants are given the drug and very closely monitored to see what side effects there are at various doses.

After the safety of the drug is shown from the phase 1 study, the medication moves into phase 2 testing. This is the stage where the effectiveness of the drug against the cancer is studied. Participation in phase 2 studies is usually offered to patients with advanced cancer who may benefit from the drug, but there is no guarantee of benefit—the clinical trial is being done to see if the drug is effective. The majority of those who take part in these trials see no improvements to their own health or disease progression and may in fact feel worse while on the experimental medication or treatment.

Phase 3 clinical trials are the ones that you may be familiar with. In this type of study, the new drug is tested against existing drugs to determine its comparative effectiveness. This is accomplished by having a control group of participants who are given a previously proven drug, against which to compare a test group of participants who are given the new drug. While a phase 3 trial is often the only way that people with cancer can have access to new drugs, there is no guarantee that they will be in the participant group that gets it. This is due to the crucial randomization process that is used to best inform health care providers about whether or not, and to what degree, a new treatment is better than those already in use.

In order to know whether one drug or treatment is better than another, it must be tested in a randomized, controlled trial. There are two concepts here that are important to understand—*randomization* and *control*. Randomization refers to the process where participants are put into one (or more) groups, purely by chance. While the actual process is complicated, simply stated, randomization is done almost as if to toss a coin—study participants have equal chances of being in either group (the one that gets the new drug, or the one that gets the current treatment). The participant does not know what group he is in and, often, his health care providers and the researchers conducting the study do not know either. This is called "blinding" and is done to prevent any bias on the part of the health care team who may be influenced if they know that the patient is getting the experimental drug or not. All participants are monitored the same while in the study.

While a control group is crucial to testing the effectiveness of a new drug, some patients don't like the idea that they may be in it—they think that they will be disadvantaged and don't want to take the risk that they are not getting the best treatment. This is a common reason why patients refuse to participate in clinical trials. If we know that the new treatment is, in fact, better, this concern would be justified, but this kind of study is only done if we are not sure which treatment is better.

There are many reasons why people agree to participate in a clinical trial. They may agree because they think this is the only way they have access to new and perhaps more effective treatment. They may trust the nurse or research assistant who talks to them about the study and they want to please them or their doctor. Some people may feel that they don't really have a choice because their cancer is no longer responding to their existing treatment (Dellson et al. 2018). Some may not understand everything they have been told and agree to participate despite this (von Itzstein et al. 2020); it is not uncommon for people to agree to participate without taking the time to think about what participation means for them (Nakada, Yoshida, and Muto 2019). They may believe that by entering the trial they get extra care. This is, in part, true because being in a clinical trial usually means extra appointments and tests.

Some people refuse to participate because they are concerned about what impact the experimental treatment may have on their health and the potential side effects (Hammer et al. There may also be hidden costs to agreeing to be part of a trial. These include the amount of time required for monitoring their response to the experimental treatment, having scans and blood tests, as well as transportation and parking costs. People who live in rural settings may be particularly burdened by having to travel long distances to participate in clinical trials (Borno et al. 2018). However, research participants are often reimbursed for travel costs; some participants receive a small amount of money or a gift card as remuneration.

The main barrier to participation is not being invited to be part of the study (Carey et al. 2017). Health care providers are often careful about who they choose to talk to about participation (Bell et al. 2020). The health care provider may consider the person's language and cultural background, family support, where they live and their ability to attend multiple extra visits to the treatment center, as well as their cognitive status. In order to consent to participate in a study, the person must be able to read and understand complex language and concepts (Schumacher et al. 2017) and be able to complete questionnaires on paper or with a computer.

There are legal and ethical requirements for anyone participating in clinical studies. These include the individual being provided with information about the procedures in the study, the risks and benefits of participating, as well as alternatives if the person decides to not participate (Glaser et al. 2020); the document is called a *consent form.* The information can be provided on paper or digitally, and the information needs to convey meaning in relatively simple terms. Most consent forms are written at a twelfth-grade education level (Somers et al. 2017); this may pose problems for those who have not completed high school or have difficulty understanding complex health information. Because of the legal requirements to provide detailed information of the procedures, risks, and benefits, it may feel overwhelming to read all the details provided in order to give truly informed consent (Simonds and Buchwald 2020). It is important to ask for clarification or explanations in simple words when helping your partner to decide whether to participate in a study or not.

Pressure from family and friends may play a role in a man's decision to take part in a clinical trial. Perhaps the family is desperate to keep him with them under any circumstances and they think that a clinical trial offers hope. They may not know all the details about the trial and think that he should be prepared to experience side effects in order to prolong his life. He may have other ideas, however, and it's important for everyone to be on the same page about what he wants and what he doesn't want.

As hard as it may be to hear that your spouse/partner does not want to take part in a clinical study, remember that this is not a rejection of *you* but rather a reflection of how he feels about his cancer and his willingness to undergo further treatment. If he is tired and doesn't want to put himself through the rigors of more treatment and additional tests, then this is his decision however difficult it is for you to accept. Keep in mind that clinical trials are often of little benefit to the participant himself but rather about finding out new treatments that may help other men, so participation is a selfless act rather than one that benefits the participant.

- ClinicalTrials.gov (http://www.clinicaltrials.gov) is a website of the National Institutes of Health that has reliable information for the public. It provides details of all the studies for different diseases, where they are located, what the study is about, and who is eligible to take part. It also provides information about whether the study is actively recruiting participants or has been completed.

- Another useful website is from the National Cancer Institute (https://www.cancer.gov/about-cancer/treatment/clinical-trials). It provides information about clinical trials, safety of participants, and what to consider when deciding about participation.
- The American Society of Clinical Oncology (https://www.cancer.net/research-and-advocacy/clinical-trials/finding-clinical-trial) also has a useful website. A helpful part of this website is a list of questions that can be asked about taking part in a clinical trial.

THE EFFECT OF PROSTATE CANCER ON COUPLES

Prostate cancer is described as a couples' cancer because of the impact of the man's cancer on the couple's relationship. A cancer diagnosis will impact any relationship, no matter what kind of cancer, but prostate cancer is seen as unique because of the impact of its treatment on the man's sexuality and sexual functioning. The impact of sexual problems after treatment affects the couple based on the premise that it is the man who drives the couple's sex life. If the man experiences sexual side effects, and he is usually or always the one who initiates sex, then the couple's sex life is assumed to decrease significantly.

Men respond to these changes in different ways. They may not recognize that their behavior has changed or that they are feeling different than usual. Their partner may not understand why their behavior has changed and may be confused as to why they are not reacting with happiness or relief when they received the "all clear" from their physician.

As you will read, over and over, in the chapters of this book, both the man and his spouse/partner need to know what the plan is for his treatment. Knowing what to expect about side effects is not only a matter of safety but also allows you, the spouse/partner, to be supportive and understanding. Some side effects of treatment are to be expected and not dangerous, while others may need immediate medical attention. Both you and your spouse/partner should know about these and what to do if something unexpected occurs.

The spouse of the man with prostate cancer may be more distressed than the man himself (Resendes and McCorkle 2006). The distress is often related to lack of information about treatment, fear of the unknown, and what will happen in the future. If the man does not include his partner/spouse in appointments and/or does not share any information he has received, his spouse's distress may impact their relationship in a negative way, and the patient may find that when he needs support, his spouse is not able to provide it due to their own emotional state. Support groups for partners acknowledge the support needed for spouses of men with prostate cancer. The website, ZERO—The End of Prostate Cancer (https://zerocancer.org/; formerly UsToo), contains valuable information for the man with prostate cancer and his loved ones and caregivers.

If you do not take care of yourself, you may get sick, depressed, or experience anxiety; this can impact the quality of support you are able to provide your spouse. One of the first signs that you are not coping well is alterations in your sleep.

Here are some tips to help with sleep:

- Go to bed at the same time each night and avoid watching TV or using devices at bedtime.
- Don't lie in bed for a long time trying to get to sleep. Get up and read a book until you feel sleepy.
- Avoid alcohol, caffeine, and large meals or snacks before bedtime.
- Get at least thirty minutes of physical exercise every day.
- Deep breathing exercises, meditation, yoga, or tai chi may help with relaxation.

The partner/spouse of a newly diagnosed man should be present for all medical appointments about treatments; it is important to hear exactly what the man has been told—relying on him to recall everything is not a good idea. Much can be lost in translation when the man reports what he heard at an appointment. This can lead to confusion and misunderstanding and may cause conflict in their relationship. Partners often feel responsible for the emotional response of the man and their own emotional health is affected. Not knowing what the plans are for treatment and/or feeling excluded from information leads to their own distress and ability to cope. Having to hide their own emotions to protect the man is also difficult and can cause distancing and avoidance in the relationship. If the partner/spouse is not included in appointments, their need for support and information about what to expect is not recognized. Family caregivers may risk their own health, physically and mentally, to support their loved one. The challenges of caregiving are many (Salifu et al. 2021); ensuring that medication is given at the right time, helping the man to move in and out of bed or up and down stairs, and being able to assess when medical care is needed can be daunting.

Women are often the searchers for and gatherers of health information for their family. This is not to suggest that men can't or don't seek out information, as many do. Looking for information can be a way to cope with a new diagnosis, but it can also be confusing and distressing. And some people choose to avoid additional information as a way of coping! There is no right or wrong way to go about this. Patients and/or their families may search the internet to find out more about their illness or the treatment offered by their health care provider. Seeking help from a librarian can also help you find online resources that are helpful.

There is, however, a lot of information on the internet that may be harmful or contains misinformation. Just because websites look professional, with nice images and testimonials from men, this does not mean that they contain accurate information. At best, they are a form of advertising and, at worst, they can be dangerous because of fraudulent claims about ineffective treatments. A study of social media and content about cancer showed that a third of the most popular websites about cancer contained misinformation, and a further third contained information that was harmful (Johnson et al. 2021).

When searching the internet for articles, it is important to make sure the websites you are using are reliable sources of information. Anyone can create a website, and any kind of information (or misinformation) can be presented on that website. It's a case of buyer beware when you surf the web. As described in chapter 3 of this book, there are a number of reliable internet sources, such as the American Cancer Society (www.cancer.org) that can be trusted.

CHANGES TO THE SEXUAL RELATIONSHIP

The treatments for prostate cancer have an impact on sexuality and masculine identity and are threatening to the man's self-image. Changes in the sexual relationship affect the man's partner, too. Interventions such as pills or devices, which help with erections, only focus on functional aspects, while the emotional fallout has a greater effect on the partner. It is not uncommon for partners to avoid talking about sexual problems. For men, erections and self-esteem are closely related, and the loss of erections poses a threat to how he sees himself. Loss of sexual function may be worse for younger men who have not yet experienced the natural decline of function related to aging.

The partner also experiences loss; the change to their sexual relationship not only impacts the overall relationship but also the partner's sense of attractiveness, when the man avoids initiating sex or doesn't respond to his partner's attempt to initiate. Most couples need support about sexual issues and strategies to improve their sex life other than advice about penetrative intercourse. Partner support is important for relationship satisfaction and this is in part dependant on the couple's communication. If the man becomes distant, the partner may blame themself for the lack of communication. This can set up further isolation for both; the man does not want to "lead them on" and/or the partner does not want to make the man feel bad, so any form of physical contact stops. The end result is a couple who lives like siblngs or college roommates, a situation that is far from optimal.

Couples who focus solely on the man achieving an erection that is sufficient for penetration say that using medications causes loss of sponteneity and what was once playful and erotic becomes medicalized, and much of the joy is absent. Adjusting to the changes in the sexual relationship takes time and it is important that the feelings of the partner are taken into account. Sexual activity for some couples is the "glue" that creates and maintains their emotional connection, and so lack of erections leads to relationship dissatisfaction or worse (Collaço et al. 2021).

There is an additional challenge for men who are on androgen deprivation therapy. In the absence of testosterone, most men lose all sexual desire as well as the ability to have erections. This may cause him shame or embarrassment and potentially reduces his quality of life. This tends to increase over time and most men will not return to their previous level of function (Donovan et al. 2018), even after they stop the treatment (Nascimento et al. 2019). The physical side effects of androgen deprivation include shrinkage of the penis and testicles, and this may exacerbate body image issues in addition to the weight gain discussed earlier (Higano 2012).

The impact of loss of desire on the couple's relationship is significant, with the absence of physical touch of any kind, feelings of isolation and loneliness for the partner, and changes in the dynamics of the relationship. Some couples may accept the loss of their sexual relationship and think that this is acceptable because the treatment is lifesaving. Other couples struggle to maintain sexual activity and eventually give up; these couples are often distressed. Finally, some couples may struggle initially and then find a way to adapt and find other ways to remain connected (Walker and Robinson 2010).

Anticipatory guidance about the effects of treatment on the man's sexuality and the impact on the partner relationship is important before starting the medication. Counselling for both the man and his partner, separately and as a couple, can be helpful in their adjustment to their new reality. Advice about non-penetrative activities may be helpful, however, for men with complete loss of libido, this is not likely going to be helpful for whom the motivation to engage in any sexual activity may be absent (Wibowo et al. 2019). Some men continue to try and please their partner sexually and this may help to maintain their emotional connection (Duthie et al. 2020).

When the couple changes their focus from erections and sexual intercourse to nonsexual touch and verbal expressions of affection and appreciation, emotional connection can be retained. Learning to adapt to changes in sexual functioning requires communication and a focus on non-penetrative sexual activites that can be as satisfying. It is also important for the couple to mourn what has been lost in order to create a new way of being sexual with each other (Wittmann et al. 2011).

DEPRESSION

Experiencing incontinence, a common side effect of prostate surgery, is associated with depression (Baden et al. 2020). Other factors include treatment regret, being younger, having a history of depression, and the recency of diagnosis (Erim et al. 2019). There are many medications used to treat depression, and consulting the man's primary care provider is the first step in accessing one of the many medications that are available.

Many people would rather try non-pharmaceutical treatments for depression, and there are a range of interventions that may be helpful.

Cognitive behavioral therapy (CBT) has been shown to be effective in treating depression (Grosse Holtforth et al. 2019). This form of psychotherapy (sometimes called "talk therapy") focuses on the person's behaviors and thoughts at the present time rather than on past issues. This may involve recognizing thoughts that create problems and reframing them, using problem-solving skills to cope with challenges, and facing fears and dealing with them instead of avoiding them. CBT can be conducted face-to-face with a therapist/counselor or via video call (Lungu et al. 2020).

Exercise is another intervention that has been shown to improve mood (Toups et al. 2017). Adding exercise to antidepressant use may be even more effective (Murri et al. 2018) and has the added benefit of improving overall health. Acupuncture may also be moderately effective in treating depression (Smith et al. 2018).

FAMILY RELATIONSHIPS

Family dynamics may become more intense after a cancer diagnosis, and adult children often do not deal well with illness in a parent. What both you and the man with prostate cancer needs is support for his and your decisions, no matter what other members of the family think or feel. Treating an adult man as if he is not making the right decision makes him feel that he has less support from his loved ones, and he may question whether they will provide him with the support that he needs during and after treatment. Offering to find information for the man is more helpful than acting as if he doesn't know what he is doing. And raised voices and demands or commands just make people defensive and angry.

COMMUNICATION

Effective communication lies at the heart of relationships. Over time, couples often stop talking to each other because they assume that they know what the other person is thinking and feeling. Unfortunately, these assumptions are most often wrong! Talking about sensitive topics such as sexuality is also often difficult; we may not have the words to explain ourselves, and very often we don't want to hurt the other person's feelings. But it is important to be able to talk about your relationship, the changes that have happened after your partner/spouse has been treated for prostate cancer, and how this has affected you.

Here are some tips that should be helpful:

- Find the right time to talk. You may need to schedule a time to lessen the risk that you catch your partner at a time when they are busy, distracted, or stressed.
- Turn off phones and other electronic devices that will derail or distract either/both of you from talking.
- Talk face-to-face. Using texts or emails is not a good idea because these are more likely to be misinterpreted.
- Use "I" statements rather than "you" statements. When you say, "You did this," or, "You are distant," the other person will naturally get defensive. This often leads to an argument and hurt feelings. Saying, "I feel like we aren't talking as much as we used to," is better than, "You've stopped talking to me."
- Be aware of your body language. Make eye contact and don't cross your arms or point a finger at the other person. An open posture, hands in your lap or at your sides, suggests that you are listening and not going to attack the other person.

When communication is not clear, misunderstandings can occur and this often leads to conflict and arguments. Some couples don't mind arguing—it may add spice to the relationship—but for others, arguments cause pain.

Four behaviors are particularly negative when arguing. These are:

- Criticism—berating your partner and accusing them of always being wrong
- Contempt—treating your partner with disrespect and disapproval
- Defensiveness—self-justifying behavior means that you are unwilling to admit the possibility that you have done something wrong
- Stonewalling—evading blame or avoiding admission about doing something wrong

If you find yourself getting angry during an argument, take a break and do something relaxing or that takes your mind off of the argument.

When you feel calmer, try to think about *why* you got so angry and then think about how to explain your behavior to your partner. And perhaps most importantly, listen to your partner. When you are angry, listening is impossible.

Letter writing allows for both of you to take some time to think about what the other person has expressed and allows each of you to be measured in your response.

Here are some tips that will hopefully encourage you to write down your thoughts and feelings:

- Initially, put your thoughts down on paper as they come into your head.
- Remember to use "I" statements!
- Leave it overnight and then reread it the next day.
- Review what you have written; highlight the points that you want to get across and then write a draft of the letter.
- Try to use supportive statements that affirm what your partner is going through and try to convey your understanding of the situation.
- Once again, take some time before rereading and editing again, if needed.
- Then, give your partner the letter . . .

There is something quite intimate about writing in your own hand. It takes longer than speech and avoids the involvement of tone and volume that often leads to an argument. Many couples write notes and letters to each other in the beginning of the relationship, but this tends to stop later on, especially in long-term relationships.

CONCLUSION

This chapter has provided you with the essential knowledge you need to support your partner/spouse from diagnosis, through treatment and beyond. Some of the content may seem technical, but these are the words you need to learn now that you are in Cancerland!

In the following chapters, you will read the stories of couples who have experienced the ups and downs, challenges and successes, growth and, for some, failure, of prostate cancer and its treatments. The couples and their stories are not real people but, rather, composites of couples

I have seen in my two decades of clinical practice. Their experiences as told in each chapter may not reflect your exact experience, or that of your partner/spouse, but there are still lessons to be learned from what happened to them and how they coped (or didn't).

I hope that you will learn something from this book. I welcome comments, questions or suggestions from anyone. I can be reached by email: drannekatz@gmail.com.

REFERENCES

Adsul, P., R. Wray, D. Boyd, N. Weaver, and S. Siddiqui. 2017. "Perceptions of urologists about the conversational elements leading to treatment decision-making among newly diagnosed prostate cancer patients." *Journal of Cancer Education* 32 (3): 580–88. doi: 10.1007/s13187-016-1025-2.

Bach, P. V., C. A. Salter, D. Katz, E. Schofield, C. J. Nelson, and J. P. Mulhall. 2019. "Arousal incontinence in men following radical prostatectomy: Prevalence, impact and predictors." *Journal of Sexual Medicine* 16 (12):1947–52. doi: 10.1016/j.jsxm.2019.09.015.

Baden, M., L. Lu, F. J. Drummond, A. Gavin, and L. Sharp. 2020. "Pain, fatigue and depression symptom cluster in survivors of prostate cancer." *Support Care Cancer* 28 (10): 4813–24. doi: 10.1007/s00520-019-05268-0.

Barocas, D. A., J. Alvarez, M. J. Resnick, T. Koyama, K. E. Hoffman, M. D. Tyson, R. Conwill, D. McCollum, M. R. Cooperberg, M. Goodman, S. Greenfield, A. S. Hamilton, M. Hashibe, S. H. Kaplan, L. E. Paddock, A. M. Stroup, X. C. Wu, and D. F. Penson. 2017. "Association between radiation therapy, surgery, or observation for localized prostate cancer and patient-reported outcomes after 3 years." *JAMA: Journal of the American Medical Association* 317 (11): 1126–40. doi: 10.1001/jama.2017.1704.

Bazinet, A., K. C. Zorn, D. Taussky, G. Delouya, and D. Liberman. 2020. "Favorable preservation of erectile function after prostate brachytherapy for localized prostate cancer." *Brachytherapy* 19 (2): 222–27. doi: 10.1016/j.brachy.2019.11.003.

Bell, J. A. H., M. T. Kelly, K. Gelmon, K. Chi, A. Ho, P. Rodney, and L. G. Balneaves. 2020. "Gatekeeping in cancer clinical trials in Canada: The ethics of recruiting the 'ideal' patient." *Cancer Medicine* 9 (12): 4107–13. doi: 10.1002/cam4.3031.

Bergner, E. M., E. K. Cornish, K. Horne, and D. M. Griffith. 2018. "A qualitative meta-synthesis examining the role of women in African American men's prostate cancer screening and treatment decision making." *Psychooncology* 27 (3): 781–90. doi: 10.1002/pon.4572.

Borno, H. T., L. Zhang, A. Siegel, E. Chang, and C. J. Ryan. 2018. "At what cost to clinical trial enrollment? A retrospective study of patient travel burden in cancer clinical trials." *Oncologist* 23 (10): 1242–49. doi: 10.1634/theoncologist.2017-0628.

Bressi, B., M. Cagliari, M. Contesini, E. Mazzini, F. A. M. Bergamaschi, A. Moscato, M. C. Bassi, and S. Costi. 2021. "Physical exercise for bone health in men with prostate cancer receiving androgen deprivation therapy: A systematic review." *Support Care Cancer* 29 (4): 1811–24. doi: 10.1007/s00520-020-05830-1.

Budaus, L., M. Bolla, A. Bossi, C. Cozzarini, J. Crook, A. Widmark, and T. Wiegel. 2012. "Functional outcomes and complications following radiation therapy for prostate cancer: a critical analysis of the literature." *European Urology* 61 (1): 112–27. doi: 10.1016/j.eururo.2011.09.027.

Capogrosso, P., and A. Salonia. 2019. "Has robotic surgery improved erectile function recovery rates in radical prostatectomy patients?" *Journal of Sexual Medicine* 16 (10): 1487–89. doi: 10.1016/j.jsxm.2019.07.029.

Carey, M., A. W. Boyes, R. Smits, J. Bryant, A. Waller, and I. Olver. 2017. "Access to clinical trials among oncology patients: Results of a cross sectional survey." *BMC Cancer* 17 (1): 653. doi: 10.1186/s12885-017-3644-3.

Chen, C., Y. Chen, L. K. Hu, C. C. Jiang, R. F. Xu, and X. Z. He. 2018. "The performance of the new prognostic grade and stage groups in conservatively treated prostate cancer." *Asian Journal of Andrology* 20 (4): 366–71. doi: 10.4103/aja.aja_5_18.

Chen, R. C. 2019. "Radiation therapy for prostate cancer: An evolving treatment modality." *Urologic Oncology* 37 (9):579–581. doi: 10.1016/j.urolonc.2019.05.023.

Cherrier, M. M., and C. S. Higano. 2020. "Impact of androgen deprivation therapy on mood, cognition, and risk for AD." *Urologic Oncology* 38 (2): 53–61. doi: 10.1016/j.urolonc.2019.01.021.

Chestnut, G. Zareba, P. Sjoberg, D. Mamoor, M. Carlsson, S. Lee, T. 2020. "Patient-reported pain, discomfort, and anxiety during magnetic resonance imaging-targeted prostate biopsy." *Canadian Urological Association Journal* 14 (5). doi: 10.5489/cuai.6102.

Collaço, N., R. Wagland, O. Alexis, A. Gavin, A. Glaser, and E. K. Watson. 2021. "The experiences and needs of couples affected by prostate cancer aged 65 and under: A qualitative study." *Journal of Cancer Survivorship* 15 (2): 358–66. doi: 10.1007/s11764-020-00936-1.

Cormie, P., and E. M. Zopf. 2020. "Exercise medicine for the management of androgen deprivation therapy-related side effects in prostate cancer." *Urologic Oncology* 38 (2): 62–70. doi: 10.1016/j.urolonc.2018.10.008.

Crawford, E. D., A. Heidenreich, N. Lawrentschuk, B. Tombal, A. C. L. Pompeo, A. Mendoza-Valdes, K. Miller, F. M. J. Debruyne, and L. Klotz. 2019.

"Androgen-targeted therapy in men with prostate cancer: Evolving practice and future considerations." *Prostate Cancer and Prostatic Diseases* 22 (1): 24–38. doi: 10.1038/s41391-018-0079-0.

Daum, L. M., E. N. Reamer, J. J. Ruterbusch, J. Liu, M. Holmes-Rovner, and J. Xu. 2017. "Patient knowledge and qualities of treatment decisions for localized prostate cancer." *Journal of the American Board of Family Medicine* 30 (3): 288–97. doi: 10.3122/jabfm.2017.03.160298.

Dellson, P., K. Nilsson, H. Jernström, and C. Carlsson. 2018. "Patients' reasoning regarding the decision to participate in clinical cancer trials: An interview study." *Trials* 19 (1): 528. doi: 10.1186/s13063-018-2916-9.

Detsky, J. S., A. F. Ghiam, A. Mamedov, K. Commisso, A. Commisso, L. Zhang, S. Liu, L. Klotz, A. Loblaw, and D. Vesprini. 2020. "Impact of biopsy compliance on outcomes for patients on active surveillance for prostate cancer." *Journal of Urology* 204 (5): 934–40. doi: 10.1097/ju.0000000000001091.

Dickinson, K. Lim, A. Kupzyk, K. 2021. "Demographic, symptom, and lifestyle factors associated with cancer-related fatigue in men with prostate cancer." *Oncology Nursing Forum* 48 (2): 423–30. doi: 10.1188/21.ONF.423-430.

Donovan, K. A., B. D. Gonzalez, A. M. Nelson, M. N. Fishman, B. Zachariah, and P. B. Jacobsen. 2018. "Effect of androgen deprivation therapy on sexual function and bother in men with prostate cancer: A controlled comparison." *Psychooncology* 27 (1): 316–24. doi: 10.1002/pon.4463.

Duthie, C. J., H. J. Calich, C. M. Rapsey, and E. Wibowo. 2020. "Maintenance of sexual activity following androgen deprivation in males." *Critical Reviews in Oncology/Hematology* 153: 103064. doi: 10.1016/j.critrevonc.2020.103064.

Edmunds, K., H. Tuffaha, D. A. Galvão, P. Scuffham, and R. U. Newton. 2020. "Incidence of the adverse effects of androgen deprivation therapy for prostate cancer: a systematic literature review." *Support Care Cancer* 28 (5): 2079–93. doi: 10.1007/s00520-019-05255-5.

El-Khatib, F., L. Huynh, M. Osman, E. Choi, F. Yafi, and T. Ahlering. 2021. "158 penile length shortening following robot-assisted radical prostatectomy: Impacts on erections and sexual bother." *Journal of Sexual Medicine* 18 (3): S86–87. doi: 10.1016/j.jsxm.2021.01.013.

Erim, D. O., J. T. Bensen, J. L. Mohler, E. T. H. Fontham, L. Song, L. Farnan, S. E. Delacroix, E. S. Peters, T. N. Erim, R. C. Chen, and B. N. Gaynes. 2019. "Prevalence and predictors of probable depression in prostate cancer survivors." *Cancer* 125 (19): 3418–27. doi: 10.1002/cncr.32338.

Fakhrejahani, F., R. A. Madan, and W. L. Dahut. 2017. "Management options for biochemically recurrent prostate cancer." *Current Treatment Options in Oncology* 18 (5): 26. doi: 10.1007/s11864-017-0462-4.

Fankhauser, C. D., M. S. Wettstein, M. Reinhardt, A. Gessendorfer, H. Mostafid, and T. Hermanns. 2020. "Indications and complications of androgen deprivation therapy." *Seminars in Oncology Nursing* 36 (4): 151042. doi: 10.1016/j.soncn.2020.151042.

Fode, M., E. C. Serefoglu, M. Albersen, and J. Sønksen. 2017. "Sexuality following radical prostatectomy: Is restoration of erectile function enough?" *Sexual Medicine Reviews* 5 (1): 110–19. doi: 10.1016/j.sxmr.2016.07.005.

Frey, A., J. Sønksen, H. Jakobsen, and M. Fode. 2014. "Prevalence and predicting factors for commonly neglected sexual side effects to radical prostatectomies: Results from a cross-sectional questionnaire-based study." *Journal of Sexual Medicine* 11 (9): 2318–26. doi: 10.1111/jsm.12624.

Geerkens, M. J. M., N. S. A. Pouwels, and H. P. Beerlage. 2020. "The effectiveness of lifestyle interventions to reduce side effects of androgen deprivation therapy for men with prostate cancer: a systematic review." *Quality of Life Research* 29 (4): 843–65. doi: 10.1007/s11136-019-02361-z.

Gentili, C., S. McClean, L. Hackshaw-McGeagh, A. Bahl, R. Persad, and D. Harcourt. 2019. "Body image issues and attitudes towards exercise amongst men undergoing androgen deprivation therapy (ADT) following diagnosis of prostate cancer." *Psychooncology* 28 (8): 1647–53. doi: 10.1002/pon.5134.

Glaser, J., S. Nouri, A. Fernandez, R. L. Sudore, D. Schillinger, M. Klein-Fedyshin, and Y. Schenker. 2020. "Interventions to improve patient comprehension in informed consent for medical and surgical procedures: An updated systematic review." *Medical Decision Making* 40 (2): 119–43. doi: 10.1177/0272989x19896348.

Gnanapragasam, V. J. 2020. "Informing informed decision-making in primary prostate cancer treatment selection." *BJU International* 125 (2): 194–96. doi: 10.1111/bju.14910.

Goldberg, H., A. E. Ahmad, T. Chandrasekar, L. Klotz, M. Emberton, M. A. Haider, S. S. Taneja, K. Arora, N. Fleshner, A. Finelli, N. Perlis, M. D. Tyson, Z. Klaassen, and C. J. D. Wallis. 2020. "Comparison of magnetic resonance imaging and transrectal ultrasound informed prostate biopsy for prostate cancer diagnosis in biopsy naïve men: A systematic review and meta-analysis." *Journal of Urology* 203 (6): 1085–93. doi: 10.1097/ju .0000000000000595.

Gonzalez, B. D., B. J. Small, M. G. Cases, N. L. Williams, M. N. Fishman, P. B. Jacobsen, and H. S. L. Jim. 2018. "Sleep disturbance in men receiving androgen deprivation therapy for prostate cancer: The role of hot flashes and nocturia." *Cancer* 124 (3): 499–506. doi: 10.1002/cncr.31024.

Gordon, B. E., R. Basak, W. R. Carpenter, D. Usinger, P. A. Godley, and R. C. Chen. 2019. "Factors influencing prostate cancer treatment decisions for African American and white men." *Cancer* 125 (10): 1693–1700. doi: 10.1002/cncr.31932.

Gordon, L., A. Dickinson, and M. Offredy. 2019. "Information in radiotherapy for men with localised prostate cancer: An integrative review." *European Journal of Cancer Care* 28 (3): e13085. doi: 10.1111/ecc.13085.

Greenberger, B. A., N. G. Zaorsky, and R. B. Den. 2020. "Comparison of radical prostatectomy versus radiation and androgen deprivation therapy strategies as primary treatment for high-risk localized prostate cancer: A systematic review and meta-analysis." *European Urology Focus* 6 (2): 404–18. doi: 10.1016/j.euf.2019.11.007.

Guan, T., S. J. Santacroce, D. G. Chen, and L. Song. 2020. "Illness uncertainty, coping, and quality of life among patients with prostate cancer." *Psychooncology* 29 (6): 1019–25. doi: 10.1002/pon.5372.

Gupta, D., K. Lee Chuy, J. C. Yang, M. Bates, M. Lombardo, and R. M. Steingart. 2018. "Cardiovascular and Metabolic Effects of Androgen-Deprivation Therapy for Prostate Cancer." *Journal of Oncology Practice* 14 (10): 580–587. doi: 10.1200/jop.18.00178.

Hammer, M. J., P. Eckardt, and M. Barton-Burke. 2016. "Informed consent: A clinical trials perspective." *Oncology Nursing Forum* 43 (6): 694–96. doi: 10.1188/16.onf.694-696.

Higano, C. S. 2012. "Sexuality and intimacy after definitive treatment and subsequent androgen deprivation therapy for prostate cancer." *Journal of Clinical Oncology* 30 (30): 3720–25. doi: 10.1200/jco.2012.41.8509.

Hoffman, K. E., D. F. Penson, Z. Zhao, L. C. Huang, R. Conwill, A. A. Laviana, D. D. Joyce, A. N. Luckenbaugh, M. Goodman, A. S. Hamilton, X. C. Wu, L. E. Paddock, A. Stroup, M. R. Cooperberg, M. Hashibe, B. B. O'Neil, S. H. Kaplan, S. Greenfield, T. Koyama, and D. A. Barocas. 2020. "Patient-reported outcomes through 5 years for active surveillance, surgery, brachytherapy, or external beam radiation with or without androgen deprivation therapy for localized prostate cancer." *JAMA: Journal of the American Medical Association* 323 (2): 149–63. doi: 10.1001/jama.2019.20675.

Hoffman, K. E., H. Skinner, T. J. Pugh, K. R. Voong, L. B. Levy, S. Choi, S. J. Frank, A. K. Lee, U. Mahmood, S. E. McGuire, P. J. Schlembach, W. Du, J. Johnson, R. J. Kudchadker, and D. A. Kuban. 2018. "Patient-reported urinary, bowel, and sexual function after hypofractionated intensity-modulated radiation therapy for prostate cancer: Results from a randomized trial." *American Journal of Clinical Oncology* 41 (6): 558–67. doi: 10.1097/coc.0000000000000325.

Holtforth, M. Grosse, T. Krieger, J. Zimmermann, D. Altenstein-Yamanaka, N. Dörig, L. Meisch, and A. M. Hayes. 2019. "A randomized-controlled trial of cognitive-behavioral therapy for depression with integrated techniques from emotion-focused and exposure therapies." *Psychotherapy Research* 29 (1): 30–44. doi: 10.1080/10503307.2017.1397796.

Imber, B. S., M. Varghese, B. Ehdaie, and D. Gorovets. 2020. "Financial toxicity associated with treatment of localized prostate cancer." *Nature Reviews Urology* 17 (1): 28–40. doi: 10.1038/s41585-019-0258-3.

Jimbo, M., M. Alom, Z. D. Pfeifer, E. S. Haile, D. A. Stephens, A. Gopalakrishna, M. J. Ziegelmann, B. R. Viers, L. W. Trost, and T. S. Kohler. 2020. "Prevalence and Predictors of climacturia and associated patient/ partner bother in patients with history of definitive therapy for prostate cancer." *Journal of Sexual Medicine* 17 (6): 1126–32. doi: 10.1016/j .jsxm.2020.02.016.

Johnson, S. B., M. Parsons, T. Dorff, M. S. Moran, J. H. Ward, S. A. Cohen, W. Akerley, J. Bauman, J. Hubbard, D. E. Spratt, C. L. Bylund, B. Swire-Thompson, T. Onega, L. D. Scherer, J. Tward, and A. Fagerlin. 2021. "Cancer misinformation and harmful information on Facebook and other social media: A brief report." *JNCI: Journal of the National Cancer Institute* djab141 doi: 10.1093/jnci/djab141.

Joseph, J. S., V. Lam, and M. I. Patel. 2019. "Preventing osteoporosis in men taking androgen deprivation therapy for prostate cancer: A systematic review and meta-analysis." *European Urology Oncology* 2 (5): 551–61. doi: 10.1016/j.euo.2018.11.001.

Jung, J. H., M. C. Risk, R. Goldfarb, B. Reddy, B. Coles, and P. Dahm. 2018. "Primary cryotherapy for localised or locally advanced prostate cancer." *Cochrane Database of Systematic Reviews* 5 (5): Cd005010. doi: 10.1002/14651858.CD005010.pub3.

Kamran, S. C., J. O. Light, and J. A. Efstathiou. 2019. "Proton versus photon-based radiation therapy for prostate cancer: Emerging evidence and considerations in the era of value-based cancer care." *Prostate Cancer and Prostatic Diseases* 22 (4): 509–21. doi: 10.1038/s41391-019-0140-7.

Khan, S., S. Thakkar, and B. Drake. 2019. "Smoking history, intensity, and duration and risk of prostate cancer recurrence among men with prostate cancer who received definitive treatment." *Annals of Epidemiology* 38: 4–10. doi: 10.1016/j.annepidem.2019.08.011.

Klaassen, Z., K. Arora, S. N. Wilson, S. A. King, R. Madi, D. E. Neal, Jr., P. Kurdyak, G. S. Kulkarni, R. W. Lewis, and M. K. Terris. 2018. "Decreasing suicide risk among patients with prostate cancer: Implications for depression, erectile dysfunction, and suicidal ideation screening." *Urologic Oncology* 36 (2): 60–66. doi: 10.1016/j.urolonc.2017.09.007.

Klotz, L. 2017. "Active surveillance for low-risk prostate cancer." *Current Opinion in Urology* 27 (3): 225–30. doi: 10.1097/mou.0000000000000393.

Klotz, T., M. Mathers, R. Klotz, and F. Sommer. 2005. "Why do patients with erectile dysfunction abandon effective therapy with sildenafil (Viagra®)?" *International Journal of Impotence Research* 17 (1): 2–4. doi: 10.1038/ sj.ijir.3901252.

Kluger, J., A. Roy, and H. H. Chao. 2020. "Androgen deprivation therapy and cognitive function in prostate cancer." *Current Oncology Reports* 22 (3): 24. doi: 10.1007/s11912-020-0884-1.

Kohaar, I., G. Petrovics, and S. Srivastava. 2019. "A rich array of prostate cancer molecular biomarkers: Opportunities and challenges." *International Journal of Molecular Sciences* 20 (8). doi: 10.3390/ijms20081813.

Kryvenko, O. N., and J. I. Epstein. 2016. "Prostate cancer grading: A decade after the 2005 modified gleason grading system." *Archives of Pathology & Laboratory Medicine* 140 (10): 1140–52. doi: 10.5858/arpa.2015-0487-SA.

Lindenberg, M. L., B. Turkbey, E. Mena, and P. L. Choyke. 2017. "Imaging locally advanced, recurrent, and metastatic prostate cancer: A review." *JAMA Oncology* 3 (10): 1415–22. doi: 10.1001/jamaoncol.2016.5840.

Lungu, A., J. J. Jun, O. Azarmanesh, Y. Leykin, and C. E. Chen. 2020. "Blended care-cognitive behavioral therapy for depression and anxiety in real-world settings: Pragmatic retrospective study." *Journal of Medical Internet Research* 22 (7): e18723. doi: 10.2196/18723.

Magee, D. E., and R. K. Singal. 2020. "Androgen deprivation therapy: Indications, methods of utilization, side effects and their management." *Canadian Journal of Urology* 27 (27 Suppl 1): 11–16.

Mallapareddi, A., J. Ruterbusch, E. Reamer, S. Eggly, and J. Xu. 2017. "Active surveillance for low-risk localized prostate cancer: What do men and their partners think?" *Family Practice* 34 (1): 90–97. doi: 10.1093/fampra/cmw123.

Manley, L., L. Gibson, N. Papa, B. K. Beharry, L. Johnson, N. Lawrentschuk, and D. M. Bolton. 2016. "Evaluation of pelvic floor muscle strength before and after robotic-assisted radical prostatectomy and early outcomes on urinary continence." *Journal of Robotic Surgery* 10 (4): 331–35. doi: 10.1007/s11701-016-0602-z.

Marzouk, K., M. Assel, B. Ehdaie, and A. Vickers. 2018. "Long-term cancer specific anxiety in men undergoing active surveillance of prostate cancer: Findings from a large prospective cohort." *Journal of Urology* 200 (6): 1250–55. doi: 10.1016/j.juro.2018.06.013.

Matta, R., A. E. Hird, E. Dvorani, R. Saskin, G. J. Nason, G. Kulkarni, R. T. Kodama, S. Herschorn, and R. K. Nam. 2020. "Rates of primary and secondary treatments for patients on active surveillance for localized prostate cancer: A population-based cohort study." *Cancer Medicine* 9 (19): 6946–53. doi: 10.1002/cam4.3341.

Matta, R., C. R. Chapple, M. Fisch, A. Heidenreich, S. Herschorn, R. T. Kodama, B. F. Koontz, D. G. Murphy, P. L. Nguyen, and R. K. Nam. 2019. "Pelvic complications after prostate cancer radiation therapy and their management: An international collaborative narrative review." *European Urology* 75 (3): 464–76. doi: 10.1016/j.eururo.2018.12.003.

Melloni, C., and M. T. Roe. 2020. "Androgen deprivation therapy and cardiovascular disease." *Urologic Oncology* 38 (2): 45–52. doi: 10.1016/j.urolonc.2019.02.010.

Merriel, S. W. D., and V. Gnanapragasam. 2019. "Prostate cancer treatment choices: The GP's role in shared decision making." *British Journal of General Practice* 69 (689): 588–89. doi: 10.3399/bjgp19X706685.

Merriel, S. W. D., D. Moon, P. Dundee, N. Corcoran, P. Carroll, A. Partin, J. A. Smith, F. Hamdy, C. Moore, P. Ost, and T. Costello. 2021. "A modified Delphi study to develop a practical guide for selecting patients with prostate cancer for active surveillance." *BMC Urology* 21 (1): 18. doi: 10.1186/s12894-021-00789-5.

Milios, J. E., T. R. Ackland, and D. J. Green. 2019. "Pelvic floor muscle training in radical prostatectomy: A randomized controlled trial of the impacts on pelvic floor muscle function and urinary incontinence." *BMC Urology* 19 (1): 116. doi: 10.1186/s12894-019-0546-5.

Mundell, N. L., R. M. Daly, H. Macpherson, and S. F. Fraser. 2017. "Cognitive decline in prostate cancer patients undergoing ADT: A potential role for exercise training." *Endocrine-Related Cancer* 24 (4): r145–55. doi: 10.1530/erc-16-0493.

Murri, M. B., P. Ekkekakis, M. Menchetti, F. Neviani, F. Trevisani, S. Tedeschi, P. M. Latessa, E. Nerozzi, G. Ermini, D. Zocchi, S. Squatrito, G. Toni, A. Cabassi, M. Neri, S. Zanetidou, and M. Amore. 2018. "Physical exercise for late-life depression: Effects on symptom dimensions and time course." *Journal of Affective Disorders* 230: 65–70. doi: 10.1016/j.jad.2018.01.004.

Nakada, H., S. Yoshida, and K. Muto. 2019. "'Tell me what you suggest, and let's do that, doctor': Patient deliberation time during informal decision-making in clinical trials." *PLOS One* 14 (1): e0211338. doi: 10.1371/journal.pone.0211338.

Nascimento, B., E. P. Miranda, L. C. Jenkins, N. Benfante, E. A. Schofield, and J. P. Mulhall. 2019. "Testosterone recovery profiles after cessation of androgen deprivation therapy for prostate cancer." *Journal of Sexual Medicine* 16 (6): 872–79. doi: 10.1016/j.jsxm.2019.03.273.

Nead, K. T., S. Sinha, and P. L. Nguyen. 2017. "Androgen deprivation therapy for prostate cancer and dementia risk: A systematic review and meta-analysis." *Prostate Cancer and Prostatic Diseases* 20 (3): 259–64. doi: 10.1038/pcan.2017.10.

Nead, K. T., S. Sinha, D. D. Yang, and P. L. Nguyen. 2017. "Association of androgen deprivation therapy and depression in the treatment of prostate cancer: A systematic review and meta-analysis." *Urologic Oncology* 35 (11): 664.e1–e9. doi: 10.1016/j.urolonc.2017.07.016.

Nelson, C. J., P. T. Scardino, J. A. Eastham, and J. P. Mulhall. 2013. "Back to baseline: Erectile function recovery after radical prostatectomy from the patients' perspective." *Journal of Sexual Medicine* 10 (6): 1636–43. doi: 10.1111/jsm.12135.

Nguyen, D. D., A. Berlin, A. G. Matthew, N. Perlis, and D. S. Elterman. 2021. "Sexual function and rehabilitation after radiation therapy for prostate cancer: A review." *International Journal of Impotence Research* 33 (4): 410–17. doi: 10.1038/s41443-020-00389-1.

Nolsøe, A. B., C. F. S. Jensen, P. B. Østergren, and M. Fode. 2021. "Neglected side effects to curative prostate cancer treatments." *International Journal of Impotence Research* 33 (4): 428–38. doi: 10.1038/s41443-020-00386-4.

Orom, H., C. Biddle, W. Underwood III, and C. J. Nelson. 2018. "Worse urinary, sexual and bowel function cause emotional distress and vice versa in men treated for prostate cancer." *Journal of Urology* 199 (6): 1464–69. doi: 10.1016/j.juro.2017.12.047.

Orom, H., C. Biddle, W. Underwood III, C. J. Nelson, and D. L. Homish. 2016. "What is a "good" treatment decision? Decisional control, knowledge, treatment decision making, and quality of life in men with clinically localized prostate cancer." *Medical Decision Making* 36 (6): 714–25. doi: 10.1177/0272989x16635633.

Owen, P. J., R. M. Daly, P. M. Livingston, and S. F. Fraser. 2017. "Lifestyle guidelines for managing adverse effects on bone health and body composition in men treated with androgen deprivation therapy for prostate cancer: An update." *Prostate Cancer and Prostatic Diseases* 20 (2): 137–45. doi: 10.1038/pcan.2016.69.

Pan, L. H., M. H. Lin, S. T. Pang, J. Wang, and W. M. Shih. 2019. "Improvement of urinary incontinence, life impact, and depression and anxiety with modified pelvic floor muscle training after radical prostatectomy." *American Journal of Men's Health* 13 (3): 1557988319851618. doi: 10.1177/1557988319851618.

Pillay, B., D. Moon, C. Love, D. Meyer, E. Ferguson, H. Crowe, N. Howard, S. Mann, and A. Wootten. 2017. "Quality of life, psychological functioning, and treatment satisfaction of men who have undergone penile prosthesis surgery following robot-assisted radical prostatectomy." *Journal of Sexual Medicine* 14 (12): 1612–20. doi: 10.1016/j.jsxm.2017.10.001.

Podder, T. K., E. T. Fredman, and R. J. Ellis. 2018. "Advances in radiotherapy for prostate cancer treatment." *Advances in Experimental Medicine and Biology* 1096: 31–47. doi: 10.1007/978-3-319-99286-0_2.

Qan'ir, Y., D. DeDeaux, P. A. Godley, D. K. Mayer, and L. Song. 2019. "Management of androgen deprivation therapy-associated hot flashes in men with prostate cancer." *Oncology Nursing Forum* 46 (4): e107–18. doi: 10.1188/19.onf.e107-e118.

Radadia, K. D., N. J. Farber, B. Shinder, C. F. Polotti, L. J. Milas, and Hsgr Tunuguntla. 2018. "Management of postradical prostatectomy urinary incontinence: A review." *Urology* 113: 13–19. doi: 10.1016/j.urology.2017.09.025.

Rancati, T., F. Palorini, C. Cozzarini, C. Fiorino, and R. Valdagni. 2017. "Understanding urinary toxicity after radiotherapy for prostate cancer: First steps forward." *Tumori* 103 (5): 395–404. doi: 10.5301/tj.5000681.

Rans, K., C. Berghen, S. Joniau, and G. De Meerleer. 2020. "Salvage radiotherapy for prostate cancer." *Clinical Oncology (The Royal College of Radiologists)* 32 (3): 156–62. doi: 10.1016/j.clon.2020.01.003.

Reamer, E., F. Yang, M. Holmes-Rovner, J. Liu, and J. Xu. 2017. "Influence of men's personality and social support on treatment decision-making for localized prostate cancer." *BioMed Research International* 2017: 1467056. doi: 10.1155/2017/1467056.

Resendes, L., and R. McCorkle. 2006. "Spousal responses to prostate cancer: An integrative review." *Cancer Investigation* 24: 192–98. doi: 10.1080/07357900500524652.

Royce, T. J., and J. A. Efstathiou. 2019. "Proton therapy for prostate cancer: A review of the rationale, evidence, and current state." *Urologic Oncology* 37 (9): 628–36. doi: 10.1016/j.urolonc.2018.11.012.

Ruane-McAteer, E., S. Porter, J. M. O'Sullivan, O. Santin, and G. Prue. 2017. "Active surveillance for favorable-risk prostate cancer: Is there a greater psychological impact than previously thought? A systematic, mixed studies literature review." *Psychooncology* 26 (10): 1411–21. doi: 10.1002/pon.4311.

Salifu, Y., K. Almack, and G. Caswell. 2021. "'My wife is my doctor at home': A qualitative study exploring the challenges of home-based palliative care in a resource-poor setting." *Palliative Medicine* 35 (1): 97–108. doi: 10.1177/0269216320951107.

Salter, C. A., P. V. Bach, E. Miranda, L. C. Jenkins, N. Benfante, E. Schofield, C. J. Nelson, and J. P. Mulhall. 2020. "Bother associated with climacturia after radical prostatectomy: Prevalence and predictors." *Journal of Sexual Medicine* 17 (4): 731–36. doi: 10.1016/j.jsxm.2019.12.016.

Salter, C. A., P. V. Bach, D. Katz, E. Schofield, C. J. Nelson, and J. P. Mulhall. 2020. "The relationship and psychosocial impact of arousal incontinence after radical prostatectomy." *Journal of Sexual Medicine* 17 (1): 94–98. doi: 10.1016/j.jsxm.2019.09.001.

Schumacher, A., W. M. Sikov, M. I. Quesenberry, H. Safran, H. Khurshid, K. M. Mitchell, and A. J. Olszewski. 2017. "Informed consent in oncology clinical trials: A Brown University Oncology Research Group prospective cross-sectional pilot study." *PLOS One* 12 (2): e0172957. doi: 10.1371/journal.pone.0172957.

Sebesta, E. M., and C. B. Anderson. 2017. "The surgical management of prostate cancer." *Seminars in Oncology* 44 (5): 347–57. doi: 10.1053/j.seminoncol.2018.01.003.

Shen, X., C. A. Pettaway, and R. C. Chen. 2020. "Active surveillance for Black men with low-risk prostate cancer." *JAMA: Journal of the American Medical Association* 324 (17): 1733–34. doi: 10.1001/jama.2020.16315.

Shevach, J., A. Weiner, and A. K. Morgans. 2019. "Quality of life–focused decision-making for prostate cancer." *Current Urology Reports* 20 (10): 57. doi: 10.1007/s11934-019-0924-2.

Siebert, A. L., L. Lapping-Carr, and A. K. Morgans. 2020. "Neuropsychiatric impact of androgen deprivation therapy in patients with prostate cancer: Current evidence and recommendations for the clinician." *European Urology Focus* 6 (6): 1170–79. doi: 10.1016/j.euf.2020.05.014.

Simonds, V. W., and D. Buchwald. 2020. "Too dense and too detailed: Evaluation of the health literacy attributes of an informed consent document." *Journal of Racial and Ethnic Health Disparities* 7 (2): 327–35. doi: 10.1007/s40615-019-00661-1.

Smith, C. A., M. Armour, M. S. Lee, L. Q. Wang, and P. J. Hay. 2018. "Acupuncture for depression." *Cochrane Database of Systematic Reviews* 3 (3): cd004046. doi: 10.1002/14651858.CD004046.pub4.

Somers, R., C. Van Staden, and F. Steffens. 2017. "Views of clinical trial participants on the readability and their understanding of informed consent documents." *AJOB Empirical Bioethics* 8 (4): 277–84. doi: 10.1080/23294515.2017.1401563.

Terrier, J. E., M. Masterson, J. P. Mulhall, and C. J. Nelson. 2018. "Decrease in intercourse satisfaction in men who recover erections after radical prostatectomy." *Journal of Sexual Medicine* 15 (8): 1133–39. doi: 10.1016/j.jsxm.2018.05.020.

Thera, R., D. T. Carr, D. G. Groot, N. Baba, and D. K. Jana. 2018. "Understanding medical decision-making in prostate cancer care." *American Journal of Men's Health* 12 (5): 1635–47. doi: 10.1177/1557988318780851.

Toups, M., T. Carmody, T. Greer, C. Rethorst, B. Grannemann, and M. H. Trivedi. 2017. "Exercise is an effective treatment for positive valence symptoms in major depression." *Journal of Affective Disorders* 209: 188–94. doi: 10.1016/j.jad.2016.08.058.

Tourinho-Barbosa, R. R., R. Sanchez-Salas, O. R. Claros, S. Collura-Merlier, A. Bakavicius, A. Carneiro, A. Stabile, M. Moschini, N. Cathala, M. Tobias-Machado, and X. Cathelineau. 2020. "Focal therapy for localized prostate cancer with either high intensity focused ultrasound or cryoablation: A single institution experience." *Journal of Urology* 203 (2): 320–30. doi: 10.1097/ju.0000000000000506.

Tunio, M. A., M. Al-Asiri, A. Al-Amro, Y. Bayoumi, and M. Fareed. 2012. "Optimal prophylactic and definitive therapy for bicalutamide-induced gynecomastia: Results of a meta-analysis." *Current Oncology* 19 (4): e280–88. doi: 10.3747/co.19.993.

van den Bergh, R. C. N., P. C. Albertsen, C. H. Bangma, S. J. Freedland, M. Graefen, A. Vickers, and H. G. van der Poel. 2013. "Timing of curative treatment for prostate cancer: A systematic review." *European Urology* 64 (2): 204–15. doi: https://doi.org/10.1016/j.eururo.2013.02.024.

van Stam, M. A., A. H. Pieterse, H. G. van der Poel, Jlhr Bosch, C. Tillier, S. Horenblas, and N. K. Aaronson. 2018. "Shared decision making in prostate cancer care—encouraging every patient to be actively involved in decision making or ensuring the patient preferred level of involvement?" *Journal of Urology* 200 (3): 582–89. doi: 10.1016/j.juro.2018.02.3091.

Varner, S., G. Lloyd, K. W. Ranby, S. Callan, C. Robertson, and I. M. Lipkus. 2019. "Illness uncertainty, partner support, and quality of life: A dyadic longitudinal investigation of couples facing prostate cancer." *Psychooncology* 28 (11): 2188–94. doi: 10.1002/pon.5205.

Verma, V., C. B. Simone, 2nd, and M. V. Mishra. 2018. "Quality of life and patient-reported outcomes following proton radiation therapy: A systematic review." *Journal of the National Cancer Institute* 110 (4). doi: 10.1093/jnci/djx208.

von Itzstein, M. S., E. Railey, M. L. Smith, C. B. White, G. W. Sledge Jr., J. R. Howell, W. Lawton, D. M. Marinucci, N. Unni, and D. E. Gerber. 2020. "Patient familiarity with, understanding of, and preferences for clinical trial endpoints and terminology." *Cancer* 126 (8): 1605–13. doi: 10.1002/cncr.32730.

Wade, J., J. Donovan, A. Lane, M. Davis, E. Walsh, D. Neal, E. Turner, R. Martin, C. Metcalfe, T. Peters, F. Hamdy, R. Kockelbergh, J. Catto, A. Paul, P. Holding, D. Rosario, H. Kynaston, E. Rowe, O. Hughes, P. Bollina, D. Gillatt, A. Doherty, V. J. Gnanapragasam, and E. Paez. 2020. "Strategies adopted by men to deal with uncertainty and anxiety when following an active surveillance/monitoring protocol for localised prostate cancer and implications for care: A longitudinal qualitative study embedded within the ProtecT trial." *BMJ Open* 10 (9): e036024. doi: 10.1136/bmjopen-2019-036024.

Walker, L. M., and J. W. Robinson. 2010. "The unique needs of couples experiencing androgen deprivation therapy for prostate cancer." *Journal of Sex & Marital Therapy* 36 (2): 154–65. doi: 10.1080/00926230903554552.

Wibowo, E., R. J. Wassersug, J. W. Robinson, A. Matthew, D. McLeod, and L. M. Walker. 2019. "How are patients with prostate cancer managing androgen deprivation therapy side effects?" *Clinical Genitourinary Cancer* 17 (3): e408–19. doi: 10.1016/j.clgc.2018.12.006.

Wilson, R. L., D. R. Taaffe, R. U. Newton, N. H. Hart, P. Lyons-Wall, and D. A. Galvão. 2021. "Using exercise and nutrition to alter fat and lean mass in men with prostate cancer receiving androgen deprivation therapy: A narrative review." *Nutrients* 13 (5). doi: 10.3390/nu13051664.

Wittmann, D., S. Foley, and R. Balon. 2011. "A biopsychosocial approach to sexual recovery after prostate cancer surgery: The role of grief and mourning." *Journal of Sex & Marital Therapy* 37. doi: 10.1080/0092623x.2011.560538.

Wu, M. L., C. S. Wang, Q. Xiao, C. H. Peng, and T. Y. Zeng. 2019. "The therapeutic effect of pelvic floor muscle exercise on urinary incontinence after radical prostatectomy: A meta-analysis." *Asian Journal of Andrology* 21 (2): 170–76. doi: 10.4103/aja.aja_89_18.

Xia, L., R. Talwar, R. R. Chelluri, T. J. Guzzo, and D. J. Lee. 2020. "Surgical delay and pathological outcomes for clinically localized high-risk prostate cancer." *JAMA Network Open* 3 (12): e2028320. doi: 10.1001/jamanetworkopen.2020.28320.

Zhu, Z., S. Zhao, Y. Liu, J. Wang, L. Luo, E. Li, C. Zhang, J. Luo, and Z. Zhao. 2018. "Risk of secondary rectal cancer and colon cancer after radiotherapy for prostate cancer: A meta-analysis." *International Journal of Colorectal Disease* 33 (9): 1149–58. doi: 10.1007/s00384-018-3114-7.

Chapter Two

Dealing with the New Diagnosis

"What Do We Do Now?"

In this chapter, a couple faces the life-changing diagnosis of prostate cancer. Like most men, no symptoms have been experienced by the man and the diagnosis comes as a shock to them both. This chapter will also explain how the diagnosis is made and common responses to it.

Brad Nolan is fifty-nine years old and has been faithfully attending annual checkups with his primary care provider, Dr. Barnes, for years. He owns a trucking company and his work is stressful. He took the company over from his dad knowing it was not an easy job; his father had died of a massive heart attack early one evening while working late, and Brad was the one who found him, slumped over his desk, hours later. So when he took charge of the company, he promised his wife, Angela, that he would be vigilant about his health. Brad visits Dr. Barnes every year in March, his birth month. So far, he has managed to keep his blood pressure in check, but at his last visit, Dr. Barnes asked him to stay for a chat after he had dressed.

Dr. Barnes had a serious look on his face when he came back to the examination room. He sat down at the small desk and turned the computer monitor so that Brad could see the screen.

"Your results from the blood tests look good, except for one thing, Brad."

Brad's heart jumped in his chest. He scanned the figures on the screen and one was red while all the others were blue.

"Your PSA is a little raised," the doctor continued, "We can repeat it in a couple of weeks but, in the meantime, I am going to refer you to a urologist."

"What does this mean, Doc?" Brad was not sure he wanted to hear the answer, but he needed to say something.

"The result is a little high, that's all. This might not mean anything, so try not to worry. We'll repeat it and if it's still raised, you'll need to see the urologist. It can take a bit of time to get an appointment with him so that's why I'm making the referral now. If the next reading is okay, we can cancel the referral."

The protein specific antigen test (PSA) is a screening test used to detect levels of a protein in the blood. An abnormal result may suggest the presence of cancer; a tissue biopsy will confirm whether cancer is present in the prostate. Men should also have a digital rectal examination (the dreaded DRE) that, when done by an experienced provider, can detect an abnormality on the posterior aspect of the prostate gland.

Brad did not say a word to Angela about the abnormal test result. She would panic and make a big fuss, and anyway, there was nothing to worry about, right? Dr Barnes was going to repeat the test in a few weeks. Brad tried to push the niggle of worry about it to the back of his mind. Work was very busy, and for, the most part, he didn't think about it until he was lying in bed at night. Angela fell asleep quickly, and her soft snores that used to ease him into sleep now kept him awake. That, and the thought of what the next test result might be. He couldn't put this out of his mind as the minutes ticked by but, eventually, he fell asleep. It was also the first thing he thought about when his alarm went off in the morning. He was tired and grumpy these mornings when he left for work, and he was very much aware that Angela was biting her tongue, not asking him what was wrong.

Three weeks later, he went to the lab and had his blood drawn for the repeat test. The young woman who did this was cheerful and it took a lot of effort not to tell her to just shut up and do her job. He was not usually a rude and angry person, but that day it felt like his life depended on the result of the blood test. One day later, at almost 6 p.m., his cell phone rang. The caller ID was blocked and, as he picked up his phone, he knew that it was Dr. Barnes calling with the news that would change his life.

"Brad?" the doctor's voice gave nothing away. "I got your results earlier today and your PSA is still a little raised. I would not worry about this if you were older, but . . ."

"What exactly does that mean, Doc?" Brad's voice was shaking and he could feel his heart hammering in his chest.

"Well, as I said when I saw you at the clinic, I want you to see a urologist who will likely want to do a biopsy. The PSA test doesn't tell us much. It could be raised for a number of reasons."

"Like what reasons? I need to know. I haven't had a decent night's sleep since I saw you and this is not helping. You need to tell me everything!"

"Calm down a minute, Brad," Dr Barnes's voice was a little louder. "If you ejaculated within forty-eight hours of having the test, it's one reason for a raised PSA or your prostate could be on the large side."

He definitely had *not* had sex or even masturbated before this last blood test, and wouldn't Dr. Barnes know if his prostate was enlarged? He had done the damn finger test, after all!

Dr. Barnes continued talking. "There's no use trying to figure this out on the phone, Brad. I sent the referral to the urologist back when I saw you and you should hear from them within a couple of days. I had my receptionist call their office to put a rush on this."

A rush? Brad was now in full panic mode. Why was there a rush? As his mind flew off in multiple directions, he heard Dr. Barnes saying goodbye but he didn't respond. He sat at his desk, the phone in his hand, his heartbeat the only sound in his ears.

Waiting for the results of blood tests is often a source of anxiety for anyone. In the case of the PSA test, many men have anxiety even when they have had the test multiple times before and the results were not suggestive of cancer. It is important to remember that this is just a screening test and not proof of cancer, but not knowing is stressful and stress can cause anxiety and depression. (Groarke et al. 2018)

Dr. Barnes's request for an urgent consultation resulted in Brad receiving a call early the next morning from the urologist's office. The person on the phone told him that he needed to have an MRI later that day and then see the urologist at the end of the week. As the person on the phone talked about what preparations he needed to do before the MRI, Brad glanced at his calendar. He had meetings the whole afternoon including an important one about a new contract that would bring in a lot of money for the company. He could not afford to miss this meeting! He interrupted the person who was still talking.

"Excuse me, can I just ask one question please?" His voice was shaking. "Can I get another appointment for this, um, MRI? I have an important meeting this afternoon that I cannot reschedule."

The person on the phone, a young woman by the sound of her voice, sounded surprised. "Mr Nolan, with all due respect, your physician asked for this appointment to be scheduled urgently."

"I know, I know, but this meeting is really important. Please can you find another time for this?"

The receptionist for the urologist was used to this. Many men tried to delay, postpone, or outright cancel their appointment. She knew they were not trying to be difficult, but it made her job so much harder. With a sigh she scanned the appointment schedule for Dr. James. She could reschedule the MRI, but it was going to be more difficult to find an opening in the urologist's busy schedule. Luckily, she found a cancellation for early the next week and rescheduled Brad's MRI.

Brad sighed with relief. "Thank you so much! I really do appreciate your efforts!"

He scribbled the dates of the appointments on a sticky note on his desk. For the rest of the day, he focused on the proposal he was going to present to get the new contract. He tried not to think about the note on his desk and, for the most part, he was successful. It was only after the meeting on his drive home that he remembered that Angela knew nothing about the rise in his PSA and the two upcoming appointments. He had to tell her, but when? He was in a good mood after the meeting that had gone well with the promise of a big new contract. He didn't want to ruin how good he was feeling. But he had to tell her.

Angela had prepared a nice dinner for them, anticipating that if his proposal was accepted for the new contract they could celebrate. If it had not gone well, then Brad would appreciate a good meal as a source of comfort. He came through the back door with a smile on his face. To Angela, it looked a little forced.

"Honey, did the meeting not go well?" Her voice reflected her concern.

"The meeting was fine," he replied, "But there's something I need to tell you."

"Do I need to open the wine now or can it wait till dinner?" Angela tried to joke with Brad but he seemed to not have heard her.

"Okay . . ." Brad took a deep breath, "There's something I haven't told you."

Angela felt a cold wave pass through her body. What was going on?

"I went to see Dr. Barnes a couple of weeks ago. He did a PSA test and it came back a bit high. He wanted me to have another test and I did it and it was still high. So now I have to see another doctor and I have to have an MRI and also a biopsy." Brad had been looking at his hands as he spoke and then he looked at Angela who had tears in her eyes.

"Why did you keep this to yourself all this time?" There was a hint of irritation in her voice.

"I don't know. I guess I didn't want you to worry, and there was a chance that the second test would be okay."

"Oh Brad, you silly, silly man." Angela put her arms around him and they stood there for a minute. She could feel his heart thumping in his chest and a shiver of fear made her hug him tightly. "It's going to be okay. It *has* to be okay. Whatever happens we'll get through this, but you have to promise me that you won't keep anything from me. I'm no fragile flower and we're in this together. Promise?"

She looked up at him as she said the last word and Brad nodded. It was his turn to have tears in his eyes and he hugged her close to him.

He went to have the MRI and realized that he had not been told what would happen while he was there. Or maybe he had been told and had not listened or heard? He wasn't aware that they were going to insert something into his rectum and he also wasn't aware that he was supposed to eat only light meals the day before and the day of the procedure. Fortunately, this did not cause a problem for the doctor doing the procedure but he was embarrassed that he had not followed the instructions.

The procedure was not painful, beyond the sensation of the endorectal coil. He had to remain very still and, while he lay there, his thoughts turned to the appointment that he would have in a few days with the urologist. His breathing quickened and he concentrated on trying to control his fear. He was surprised to hear a voice coming from the speaker near his head telling him that the procedure was over and that he could move and would be allowed out of the machine in a few minutes.

Magnetic resonance imaging (MRI) is increasingly being used to identify the extent of prostate cancer and if it has spread outside the prostate. The images are clearer and more detailed than other kinds of scans.

Brad saw the urologist, Dr. James, the next week. He was a tall man who looked to be in his late sixties. He was balding and had a slight stoop, as if he had spent a lot of time bent over, examining men. This was probably true, thought Brad as the doctor did a very extensive examination of his prostate. When he was dressed, Dr. James came back into the room, carrying a laptop.

"Let me show you the MRI scan," he said as he sat down on a rolling stool and pushed himself next to Brad. "This here," he pointed to something on the screen, "This here is a suspicious lesion. The radiologist has given it a PI-RADS score of 4 which means that it is very likely cancer. You're going to need to have a biopsy and my assistant will come and explain everything to you." He shook Brad's hand and left the room, leaving the door slightly open.

Brad was stunned; he didn't know what to think and his impulse was to get out of there as quickly as possible. He started to get out of the chair but before he could stand up, Dr. James's assistant entered the room.

"How ya doing . . ." the man looked at a piece of paper in his hand, ". . . Brad?"

"How do you think I'm doing?" Brad's voice was louder than he intended.

"I'm sorry," replied the assistant, "Just trying to keep it light here. Dr. James is going to do a biopsy on you a little later this week. The booking person is just confirming the time. I have some things we need to talk about. Oh, by the way my name is Jared."

Brad glared at the assistant, who seemed oblivious to his stare.

"So here's some info about what to expect when you have the biopsy. There's also a prescription for an antibiotic that you need to take the day before and the day of . . . um . . . any questions?"

Brad shook his head. This person was annoying him and he needed to get out before he said something he'd regret. On his way out of the clinic, the receptionist gave him another piece of paper with the appointment for the biopsy. He pushed it into his pocket, not caring that it was now crumpled. He sat in his car for a few minutes, not sure that he could drive just yet. He needed to go back to the office, but he was not sure that he would be able to focus on anything. He called his secretary who told him that he didn't have any meetings that afternoon, so he called Angela to see if she was at home.

"I was just about to go and get groceries," she said, "What's wrong? You sound awful."

"I was just at the urologist. . . . I have to have a biopsy."

"Okay . . . what does that mean?" Angela could hear the panic in her husband's voice.

Brad realized that he didn't know what to tell her. He couldn't recall what the doctor's assistant had told him. He has thrown the papers he was given on the seat of his car but then he remembered the piece of paper in his pocket that the receptionist had given him.

"Hand on a second, Ang, I've got a piece of paper here." He pulled the crumpled paper out of his pocket and read what it said to his wife. "Okay, the appointment for the biopsy is . . . oh no! It's for *this* Friday! That's way too soon!"

"Brad, honey, take a deep breath. Where are you now?" Angela tried to calm her husband.

"I'm in the parking lot of the clinic! I'm coming home now! Wait for me at the house!"

Angela heard the click as Brad's phone switched to the car speakers and then she heard the engine start and then nothing. Brad had cancelled the call and was now probably speeding home.

She was waiting for him in the garage and hugged him as he got out of the car. He gave her the papers that the urologist's assistant had given him, and she sat at the kitchen table, reading the instructions as he paced the floor.

"Brad, you can do this. This biopsy will confirm whether you have cancer or not. I understand this is tough, but we need to know! We can't be in this 'no man's land' of something showing on the MRI but not being sure what it is."

Brad nodded his head. He really didn't like the idea of having the biopsy and he didn't really know what was involved. He had not read the instructions and he hadn't really heard what that Jared person had said. He sighed as he went to the fridge to get a beer; he deserved one after what he had been through even though it was only 2 p.m.

The images from the MRI can be used to guide the prostate biopsy. Because the images are so detailed, the person performing the biopsy can take tissue samples from any area(s) of concern. This is called an MRI-fusion biopsy.

Men are also likely to experience significant anxiety as they wait for the results of the biopsy. This may affect their sleep and ability to function normally.

Brad had the biopsy and, while it was not excruciating, it was certainly not pleasant. He was warned by the urologist's assistant that he might have some blood in his urine for days or even weeks afterward, and his ejaculate might also contain some old blood and be discolored. He was not sure how he was going to manage his anxiety for the next week as he waited for the results of the biopsy.

Angela was sympathetic when she picked him up after the procedure. He had thought that he could drive himself there and then go back to the office, but he was glad that she had insisted on driving him. He did not feel really bad, just exhausted and a little sore as the local anesthetic wore off. He did some work in the afternoon in his home office and went to bed early. He was dreading the next appointment with Dr. James, when he would get the results of the biopsy. Angela told him in no uncertain terms that she was coming with him to that appointment. He was reluctant, because it might look like he couldn't handle things on his own, but she told him to get over himself and she was coming with—no ifs, ands, or buts about it! He was secretly pleased that she was going to go with him; she could listen to what the doctor said and, based on his lack of recall from the other appointments, this was a good thing.

The day of the appointment came, and, by this time, Brad just wanted to know for sure what the future held. He was not able to concentrate well at work and even though he tried to pretend that nothing was wrong, his secretary kept asking if he was okay. He tried to avoid snapping at her; she was just looking out for him, but he could not share this with anyone.

Dr. James was running late, and sitting in the now-full waiting room was difficult. Angela held his hand and he tried to keep calm, but his heart was racing and he was breathing fast. Eventually, almost forty minutes past his appointment time, he was ushered into the doctor's office. They sat there for another ten minutes until Dr. James entered the room, the door banging closed behind him.

"Sorry, folks," Dr. James spoke loudly as he sat down behind his desk and started typing on the computer. "Okay, here are the results of your biopsy."

Brad could feel himself holding his breath.

"Unfortunately, the biopsy confirmed the findings on the MRI. You have prostate cancer, but there's no need to panic."

Brad blinked; no need to panic? He had *cancer*.

"The biopsy showed that six of the samples we took had cancer in them. It is moderately aggressive and you should have treatment. Jared, my assistant, will talk to you about this and give you more information. I'm sorry that I have to rush off. I have surgery this afternoon and have to clear out the waiting room."

Brad and Angela looked at each other. That was it? They were both in shock; first, that Brad had cancer, and second, that the urologist had not even taken the time to ask if they had any questions! There was a knock at the door and Jared, the doctor's assistant, entered the room.

"Hello again, Brad." He put out his hand toward Angela and introduced himself. "I wish we could have met under better circumstances, but here we are."

"I'm Angela, Brad's wife. This has not been a good day."

"I'm sorry that Dr. James had to rush off. It's been a crazy day here. But I am here to answer your questions and to explain things if you are interested."

"Damn straight we need an explanation!" Brad did not try to hide his irritation. Angela held his hand even tighter than before and cleared her throat.

"My husband is upset, and I am too. The doctor didn't explain anything, and frankly, I didn't hear much after he told us that Brad has cancer." Angela was trying not to cry but she was fighting a losing battle.

"Okay, I am going to explain everything to you. Do you need some water before I start?"

The couple shook their heads; they wanted more information, and they wanted it now!

"As I hope Dr. James told you, there were six out of the twelve cores that contained cancer. One of the samples, or cores, was taken from the lesion that was identified on the MRI. We base the aggressiveness of the cancer on the Gleason score, and in your case, there were three cores that were graded as Gleason 6, and the other three were Gleason 7. I'll explain the details of this in a minute. Do you have any questions at this point?"

Once again, they shook their heads.

Jared went on to explain what the Gleason score meant. He spoke slowly and stopped often to allow them to ask questions. Despite Brad's initial irritation with the young man, Jared was good at explaining things, and Brad found himself listening intently.

The Gleason score is a measure of the aggressiveness of the prostate cancer. Scores are reported in numbers or as a group, as explained in chapter 1.

Neither Brad nor Angela had any questions; they looked like deer caught in the headlights.

"It's a lot of information, I know," said Jared with a small smile. "Is there anything that was confusing or something that you want me to go over with you?"

Angela felt like her head was going to explode. "I need time to figure this out. Do you have anything in writing that we can take home to read over?"

"Of course, Mrs. . . . um . . . Angela. Let me go and put a package together for you and, while I do that, perhaps you will think of some questions."

Angela looked at Brad and she could see the confusion on his face. She reached over and took his hand. "We'll get through this, honey, you know we will. I think we just need to go home and think about what Jared has told us. And maybe you, I mean we, should also talk to Dr. Barnes about this. Maybe he can help us understand more about what this means."

Brad nodded. He wanted to leave the clinic and never come back.

Jared returned with a folder under his arm and a few documents in his hand. He handed the folder to Angela and once again sat down on a stool next to the couple. "This here is your biopsy report, Brad. Would you like me to explain the results to you before you leave?"

They both answered at the same time.

"Yes, please," said Angela.

"No, thanks," said Brad.

"Okay, so it's one all!" Jared smiled at them and Angela smiled back, but Brad just glared. "This will only take a minute, and I think you'll find it useful." Jared's voice was firm. He had seen this before with other men. "Based on the results of the biopsy, you have intermediate prostate cancer with moderate volume. You have 6 out of 12 cores that were positive for cancer. Three of them were Gleason $3 + 4 = 7$ and 3 were Gleason $3 + 3 = 6$. This is good news, as it means that the cancer is likely confined to the prostate, and all of the treatments we can offer you will control the cancer. Do you have any questions?"

Brad got up to leave. He didn't care if he was being rude, but he really needed to get out of there. Jared's explanation had not helped him at all. If anything, he was more confused than ever.

Angela got up to follow him. She turned to Jared and asked if they could talk to him on another occasion.

"Of course, here's my card. You can call me anytime, and I will answer any questions or even make an appointment to see you." Jared could see that Angela was struggling to control her emotions. It didn't help that Brad had left the room without her.

Angela caught up with Brad in the lobby. He was standing at the revolving door with his arms crossed, looking back at her as she walked as fast as she could toward him. She had the folder that Jared had given her and the paper with the biopsy results in her hand.

"Brad!" Angela could not control how annoyed she was with him, "You left without me! I understand that you're upset, but that was plain rude of you!"

Brad started to respond to her but then his shoulders dropped and he looked like someone had punched him in the stomach. "I'm sorry honey. I just had to get out of there! It's too much! I couldn't handle it anymore!"

Angela took his arm and looked at him, her expression showing him that she understood. "Let's go home. We don't have to talk about this now. When you're ready, just tell me and we can try and sort this out."

Everyone's response to a cancer diagnosis is different. Some people want to hear all the details while others need to take time to allow the news to sink in. The response of the man's partner is also unique. Some partners are very involved in all aspects of the diagnosis, from discussing the man's PSA test results to giving an opinion about the need for a biopsy.

Brad was silent on the way home. He drove too fast, but Angela kept quiet. She didn't want to set him off, so she closed her eyes, breathed in and out slowly, and prayed that nothing bad would happen. When they arrived home, Brad went straight to his home office, shut the door, and remained there for the rest of the afternoon. Angela felt helpless, and she didn't like that. She had always been sure of herself and the decisions she had made. At the start of their relationship, she and Brad had talked about having children; she was firm in her decision to not have any. Her childhood had been traumatic, and she was scared that she would turn into her mother, who had treated her so badly. Brad was disappointed; he came from a big family and, as the oldest of six kids, he wanted to have lots of children. But she was clear; if Brad wanted to marry her, he had to be okay with not having children.

She took out her laptop and googled "prostate cancer." Before she knew it, three hours had gone by, and she had not moved. It was close to dinnertime and she had not prepared anything. Brad was still in his home office, and she was hungry. She knocked on the door and asked him if he wanted something to eat. He opened the door, and Angela reached out to hug him. He looked so defeated that she felt guilty that she had been irritated with him on the drive home.

"I didn't take out anything for dinner but we have some cheese and crackers and I think a nice bottle of wine might just be what the doctor . . . nope. Not going to say that!"

Brad smiled at her. Nothing that the doctor ordered would be good right now, and he knew that she was thinking the exact same thing.

They sat outside on the deck. The white wine in the glasses glowed in the evening light. The cheese and crackers had been a good choice, and Angela had found some olives in the back of the fridge.

"Honey, it may be too soon, but I found some interesting information on the internet." Angela was cautious in her approach about the information she had found on Google that afternoon.

Brad sighed. He had had enough information that morning from Jared. But he trusted Angela, and if she thought she had found something of value, then he was willing to listen. "Okay . . . what did you find?"

"Well, there seems to be some interesting stuff on biomarkers."

"And what are they?" Despite his best efforts he grew irritated. He did not use computers for anything other than checking the stock market and for some things at work. He didn't trust the internet and, while Angela was always looking up something or reading stuff, he preferred the local daily newspaper and news on TV.

Angela kept her voice under control, but now she was irritated. Brad acted like he was eighty-nine rather than fifty-nine about some things, and the internet was the biggest of these. "Just listen and try not to judge, please! What I read says that these biomarkers can be helpful to guide men with prostate cancer in their decision-making. That's all. Jared didn't mention them and I think we should ask Dr. James about it when you see him the next time. When are you going to see him again?"

Brad shrugged. He was not sure he wanted to see anyone, especially Dr. James, any time soon. Angela was quiet as she tried to remember if Jared had said anything about another appointment. She could not recall anything, and she had read every page in the folder that she had been given. Now what were they supposed to do?

Many people turn to the internet for health information. It is important to use sources that are valid and trustworthy. Websites such as the American Cancer Society (www.cancer.org) and the American Urological Association (www.auanet.org) provide good information and advice. But caution should be applied to any website that promotes a single medication or treatment, as these are usually trying to sell you something that has not been tested or may not be safe.

The next morning, Angela called the clinic and was put through to Jared. He apologized profusely that he had let them leave without notification of Brad's next appointment with Dr. James. He told her the date; it was exactly a week away.

"It's the last appointment of the day so that Dr. James has time to answer all your questions and also to talk to you about what comes next."

Angela was not sure what he meant. "What comes next" sounded ominous.

"Please don't be alarmed!" Jared tried to reassure her. "Dr. James likes his patients to be fully informed about treatment options. I'll be there if you want, and I can stay as late as you need to be sure that you understand everything."

Angela told Brad about the upcoming appointment.

"What if I don't go?" Brad was not joking. His impulse was to ignore the whole thing and just wait it out.

"Brad," Angela's voice was cold as steel. "You *will* go, and I will be with you. You do not have a choice. We are *not* going to talk about this anymore. Got it?"

Now Brad looked embarrassed. There were certain things that he did not want to talk about, his health being the main one. Ever since his dad had died, Angela had been like a bear when it came to him getting regular checkups. "Okay, okay." One thing he knew was when to give up.

The next week they went back to Dr. James's clinic, and this time he was not running late or in a hurry. He went over Brad's biopsy results and explained exactly what Jared had told them. This time, Brad was able to hear what was being said, and he had a lot of questions. Angela had written out her questions and she didn't interrupt the doctor. She waited patiently until he had finished talking, but before she could ask the first of her questions, Brad jumped in.

"How did this happen? I'm not even sixty yet! And no one in my family has had cancer! Not even one person!"

"Your biggest risk factor is that you are a male and you have a prostate," Dr. James had said these words so many times. "But the most important thing, moving forward, is for you to start thinking about what treatment you want to have."

Before Brad could say anything, Angela raised her hand. "Excuse me, Dr. James, but I have a question. I read about biomarkers. Why haven't you tested for these? Or have you?"

Dr. James cleared his throat. This was another topic that patients were asking about more and more frequently. "We currently don't have enough evidence that biomarkers add anything to the diagnosis, but this may change over the next few years. But there are some tests available right now if you want to pay for them. I am not using them routinely but, certainly, you have the right to request one."

The urologist didn't sound convinced that this was a good idea, and neither was Brad, so he declined.

Dr. James did not seem to be in a hurry. He had loosened his tie and he seemed almost relaxed. Jared had been sitting quietly against the wall and he, too, seemed at ease. Brad was confused by this. His life was in their hands, and they didn't seem perturbed at all!

Angela was sitting close to him, and she could feel him trembling. She put her hand on his arm and squeezed. "Okay, so one more question, if I may . . ."

"Go ahead, Angela," replied Jared.

"What do we do now?" Her voice was a little too loud, but she was concerned that the two professionals in the room were too calm. This was her husband, and he had cancer! Dr. James had not told them anything about treatment and she had a long list of questions about that.

"That's another conversation for another day," Dr James replied. "Jared will give you more information at the end of our meeting and then you take your time in deciding about treatment."

Brad and Angela looked at each other and then at Jared. What was the doctor talking about? How could they make a decision? They are, or rather, Brad was the patient and shouldn't the professionals tell them what to do?

Jared could see their confusion. "I'm going to meet with you again once you've had the opportunity to read the material that I'm going to give you. I know this feels like a protracted process, but it's very important that you take the time to consider all your options. And you *do* have options, Brad, and you also have time to make a decision."

Jared's calm voice was reassuring for Angela, but Brad looked like he was irritated again. Angela did not want a repeat of their previous visit where he stormed out of the office.

"Okay. So we have some sort of plan. Jared, can we meet sooner rather than later? We need to move forward with this. You said we have time but we, I mean, I don't want this to drag on. Am I right, honey?"

She looked at Brad, who nodded his head in agreement. He wanted to get out of there *now*.

Jared excused himself and the couple were left with Dr. Barnes, who was looking at something on his computer. He seemed immersed in whatever he was doing and did not notice when they got up and left the room. How strange, thought Angela as they headed for the lobby. She had to walk fast to keep up with Brad and they almost missed Jared, who was coming out of another office with a package in his hands. She had never felt so scared in her life, but she knew that she had to face what came next.

CONCLUSION

The diagnosis of any cancer comes as a shock and for men diagnosed with prostate cancer; the shock is exacerbated by the lack of symptoms that is common with this cancer. As you will see in chapter 3, all treatments will affect the man's quality of life and so deciding about treatment is not easy. The partner of the man with prostate cancer plays an important role in supporting the man as well as in searching for and understanding the information necessary for treatment choice. The partner often has to put their own feelings aside as they provide support and educate both themselves and the newly diagnosed man.

Reflective Questions

After reading this chapter:

- How do you cope with the news of the cancer diagnosis in your husband/partner while, at the same time, helping him to adjust to the diagnosis?
- What might help the situation if the man doesn't want to deal with the diagnosis and seems to prefer to leave his partner to deal with everything?
- How can you assess if the information you find on the internet is reliable?

For more information about prostate biopsies: https://www.radiology info.org/en/info/prostate-biopsy

REFERENCES

Groarke, A., R. Curtis, D. M. J. Walsh, and F. J. Sullivan. 2018. "What predicts emotional response in men awaiting prostate biopsy?" *BMC Urology* 18 (1): 27. doi: 10.1186/s12894-018-0340-9.

Chapter Three

Treatment Decision-Making
"Is This the Right Treatment?"

The process of choosing a treatment can be confusing. Because men with localized prostate cancer have options for treatment (see chapters 4 to 6), they are asked to pick the one they think is best for them. This is not easy, and the partner is often asked for their opinion. In this chapter, you will meet a couple who have different views on what treatment the man should have. This has the potential to cause conflict and to negatively impact the couple when the need for love and support is very high.

Walter and Renee Humphreys have been married for fifty years and now face the biggest challenge they have ever encountered. Walter was a police officer until he retired sixteen years ago, and since then, he has kept himself busy playing checkers with his retired friends, supervising their three grandsons, who are now in high school, and growing vegetables in a small plot he rented in a community garden. Renee is a retired daycare worker who is very involved in her church with various activities and charity work. They moved from their house in the suburbs when Walter retired and now live in a fifty-five-plus complex with mostly other African American tenants. They have made good friends and they now have a better social life than they did when they were younger.

Like many men his age—seventy-six years old—he went to the bathroom multiple times a night. He wasn't quiet about it either; he left the bathroom door open after turning on the light, and this woke Renee.

After arguing about this for months, he finally saw a urologist, who ordered a PSA test and scheduled him for the "rotor rooter" procedure, where tissue was scraped from his prostate gland to allow for full bladder emptying. They found cancer in the tissue that was removed from the prostate and, after a biopsy, he was diagnosed with prostate cancer.

He barely mentioned having a biopsy to Renee; this was "men's" business as far as he was concerned. He told her he was having some tests and when he came back from the appointment with the urologist, he just said that they had found "something" on his prostate. Renee pressed him about what the "something" was and eventually he told her it was cancer. When she heard the word "cancer" she felt like her heart was going to stop.

Their marriage has not always been easy; Walter has firm ideas about male and female roles, and these are very different from Renee's. They have one son, Benjamin, who is now forty-eight years old and married, with three teenage sons. Walter had wanted a large family, but Renee decided when Benjamin was three years old that he would be their one and only. Walter worked long shifts as a police officer, and in her opinion, she had the sole responsibility of raising their son. Money was often tight, and she needed to work to support them; having another child was just not possible under those circumstances. In her heart, she knew that Walter has never really forgiven her for this.

Walter has always been physically active and even though he was no longer required to keep fit, he took pride in wearing the same size pants he did before he retired. Renee was diagnosed with diabetes in her fifties and controlled her blood sugar levels with a strict diet; this is probably why Walter had not put on weight over all the years, she often reminded him. Walter didn't have a family history of any kind of cancer, and neither of them had a good understanding of medical matters. Benjamin, their son, is a paramedic, and as soon as they heard about Walter's cancer, they appointed him as the expert in these things. Benjamin was not comfortable with this; like many adult children, he saw his father as invincible and someone who would live forever. His father's diagnosis had shaken him to the core, and he felt helpless to support his parents.

Renee brought up the topic of surgery for his cancer on a weekly basis. This happened most often on Sundays, after she returned from church. The pastor, Reverend Blake, called for prayers for the sick just before the end of the service. As she bowed her head in prayer, she was reminded again that her husband had cancer and was not doing anything about it. She would raise the topic as they ate lunch and every week Walter would get annoyed.

"Renee, I do not want to talk about this. And I especially don't want to talk about it when I'm eating! You have prepared a delicious meal for us, as you do every Sunday, and every Sunday you ruin it by bringing up this subject! When are you going to cease and desist?"

His voice was raised, and she imagined that this is how he used to talk to the people he arrested. He had always managed to keep his police work and his home life separated when he was still working, and it was only when he was annoyed that his "police" voice made an appearance, even now, sixteen years later. But she was scared that while he waited, the cancer was spreading and she could lose him. Just the thought of this made her feel cold all over.

"But Walter, dearest, I'm scared that . . ." She could barely say the words. "I'm scared that if you don't do something, well . . . I'm scared!"

It is not uncommon for couples to have different ideas about treatment for prostate cancer. For many people, the initial reaction to a diagnosis of cancer is to "get it out" and as soon as possible. The partner of the man may feel exactly the same way and encourage him to have surgery as soon as possible But some men need to take time deciding what treatment they are going to have, particularly when there are choices about treatment as there often are in prostate cancer.

Benjamin came to visit later that afternoon with two of his three teenage boys. Walter was thrilled to see them as always, and he and the boys went for a walk to a nearby park where they could throw a football around without risking a neighbor's windows. While they were gone, Renee used her time alone with Benjamin to talk about his father.

"I'm at my wit's end with that man!" she said, realizing as the words left her mouth that their son usually got defensive if she spoke ill of his father.

"Mom, please . . ." Benjamin replied as she knew he would.

"But, Benjamin! He has *cancer*, and he won't do anything about it! This is madness! I don't know what's got into him!"

"Mom! Getting mad at him won't help! He needs to take the time he needs to decide. What am I supposed to do?"

Renee sighed. Walter had insisted on going to his next appointment by himself. When he came back, he didn't say much. She knew that nagging him to tell her what he learned was a recipe for an argument so she didn't ask him other than "how did the appointment go?" Her only hope lay with Benjamin; he was a paramedic and the next closest thing to a doctor in her mind.

"Benjamin! You must know about this! You went to school to study all this!"

"Mom! I went to school thirty years ago! And I'm a paramedic, not a cancer doctor! I know about heart attacks and strokes and overdoses! This is way out of my league!"

Renee sighed again. What was she going to do? She had prayed about this, but it didn't seem to be making any difference to her husband. He still had not had any treatment and it was now three months since he was told about the cancer. Then she had an idea.

"Maybe WE can go and talk to his doctor!" She smiled at her son, pleased with herself for thinking about this. "If I don't understand something then you can explain it to me later!"

Benjamin forced himself to not roll his eyes. There were times when he was shocked by his mother's lack of knowledge. He quickly reminded himself that she was almost seventy-five years old and had no education beyond eighth grade, and this was not her fault. He knew from experience that doctors often talked above patients' understanding; this had frustrated him numerous times when accompanying a patient to the ER. He understood that his mother needed help, but how was he supposed to do that?

The ability of a person to access, understand, and act on medical information to make health care decisions is called health literacy. People's reading, writing, and number skills are part of health literacy, but medical terms and procedures are complicated and pose a challenge to many ordinary people.

Benjamin sat silently for a few minutes. His heart ached as he thought about how difficult this was for his mother. She had always been there for him, much more than his father, who was often at work when Benjamin needed help with something. His relationship with his father had not always been a good one; his father was a hard taskmaster who treated his son like a potential troublemaker. While his father didn't bring his policing work home, he certainly brought his policing attitude to his interactions with his son. Benjamin hadn't really realized this until he became a father and had to deal with three young and energetic boys. It was not easy, and his admiration for his mother had grown even greater over the past years. He loved his parents, and he knew that he had to help them as they negotiated this new challenge.

"Okay, Mom. I'll come with you to see Dad's doctor, but Dad has to come too. It's not fair to him if we go without him, and he needs to hear the same information."

Renee nodded. She wasn't sure what her husband would say to this idea and she was a little scared to ask him. "Would you talk to Dad about this? Please, Benjamin. He thinks I'm a nag whenever I try to talk to him."

Benjamin nodded his head. "I'll try and see if he's still at the park with the boys. Maybe we can talk on the way back."

Renee gave him a grateful smile as he got up from the kitchen table and headed to the door. He loved her so much and would do almost anything for her. He met his father and his boys as they were rounding the corner on the street toward home. The boys were a few feet behind his father, looking at their phones and laughing at something. His father was carrying the football and had an irritated look on his face.

"What is wrong with young people these days?" he grumbled as Benjamin approached him. "All they could manage was thirty minutes throwing the ball around and then they needed to check on something on their phones! What could be so important?"

Benjamin shrugged his shoulders and smiled; he had thought the same thing multiple times. He was glad that his boys were occupied as he really wanted to talk to his father about going with him to the doctor, and walking would mean they wouldn't have to make eye contact.

He cleared his throat. "Um, Dad. I was wondering if Mom and I could come with you to the doctor? There's some stuff that I need to know, and, well, Mom seems really worried about you."

"Did your mother put you up to this, boy?" Benjamin felt himself shrink at the anger in his father's voice. It was always like this; his father's anger made him feel like he was six years old again. His mother's worried face flashed across his brain.

"Dad, you can't be angry with Mom. She loves you, and she's worried about you. And honestly, I am too. I don't understand why you're not getting the surgery. I don't know what the doctor said to you, and you seem to be treating this as a big secret. That's not fair to Mom, and it's not fair to the rest of your family. Think about your grandsons." Benjamin turned to look at his sons, who were now even farther back, engrossed in doing something with their phones. He looked at his father who had also turned to look at the boys. They shared a smile and a shrug, the two men suddenly aware how similar they were now.

"Ah, Benjamin," Walter started to talk to his grown son, "I'm not hiding anything, at least not deliberately. I just need time to think about things. The doctor, he wants me to have surgery, but I'm just not sure. You know what they're like . . . they talk, talk, talk . . . and half the time, no . . . more than that, I don't know what the hell . . . I mean heck, they're going on about. I think they just want to take my money and don't really care about what I want!"

Benjamin said nothing. Some of what his father had said made sense to him. He avoided going to the doctor himself and he certainly had heard stories about how other African American people were treated by some of the doctors he knew at various hospitals.

"Dad? Did the doctor treat you badly?" Benjamin could feel his heart beating a little faster.

"No, no! The last time I saw him he just talked over my head, is all. I didn't really hear much after the cancer word, you know. And then when I went back, I didn't see him at all. I saw this nice girl, but I can't remember her name. Anyway, she talked to me about the surgery, but I don't know if I want to do that! She told me stuff that really scared me . . . wetting myself and some other stuff I don't want to talk about. She gave me things, pamphlets, to read but I can't remember where I put them."

Benjamin sighed. It seemed to him like his parents really needed his help or at least the little help he could offer. And he also needed to talk to some of the doctors that he knew from work. He hung out with a couple of the ER doctors; they played basketball once a month and then went out for beers. Maybe they could help.

African American men are 70 percent more likely to be diagnosed with prostate cancer than their Caucasian counterparts (Siegel 2020); they are also twice as likely to die of their cancer. Factors such as racial disparities play a role in this (Airhihenbuwa and Liburd 2006; Williams and Rucker 2000) as do income, health insurance, and education. Historical mistrust of the health care system is common in African Americans (Vapiwala et al. 2021) and has an impact on cancer screening.

Walter reluctantly agreed to another appointment with the urologist, and Renee organized this. It wasn't easy finding a time that Benjamin could go with them due to his shift work, but she finally found a time that worked for him. She was nervous to meet this doctor, and she dressed in her church best. Walter shook his head as she arranged the hat on her head.

"Renee," he said in a firm voice, "No need for that. It's a doctor's appointment and not a meeting with the First Lady."

She reluctantly removed the hat and put it away carefully in its box. Now she had to fix her hair and if she didn't hurry, they would be late.

Walter drove slowly to the urologist's office. Benjamin's car was already in the parking lot, and he was leaning against the car door, looking at his watch.

"Do not say a word," Walter was more gruff than usual, "It's your mother's fault. She was going to wear a damn hat!"

Benjamin did not reply, but he smiled at his mother and put his arm around her shoulders. They waited a good ten minutes before they were escorted to the doctor's office. Benjamin looked around with interest. The chairs were covered in brown leather and there were oil paintings on the wall, mostly of horses and country scenes. Before he could explore more, a short man wearing a well-fitted suit entered the room and sat down at the desk.

"Walter, nice to see you again. And who have you brought with you today?"

The man hadn't introduced himself, so Benjamin put out his hand. "You are?" he asked.

"Oh. Sorry folks. I thought you knew. I'm Dr. Settler. I'm Walter's urologist. How can I help you today?"

Benjamin tried to hide his irritation. "I'm Benjamin Humphreys, my father is Walter. This is my mother, Mrs. Renee Humphreys."

"Nice to meet you all. So, Walter . . . have you finally decided to have the surgery?"

Walter was sitting in one of the brown leather chairs, looking at his hands in his lap. Before he could answer, there was a soft knock on the door and a young woman's head appeared.

"Oh, here's Julie!" Dr. Settler seemed relieved to see her. "Julie, these are the Humphreys. You met Walter a while ago. Walter is here with his family today and I thought you could do the pre-op teaching after he signs consent for the surgery."

Walter looked up. This was definitely not going the way he thought it would. Before he could say anything, his wife cleared her throat.

"Dr. ummm, Settler?" she seemed unsure if she had his name right, "We are here to get more information about what is wrong with Walter. Our son Benjamin? He's a paramedic."

Benjamin stifled a groan. Why did she have to tell him that?

Julie interrupted and reached over to shake Walter's hand. "Nice to see you again Mr. Humphreys. And nice to meet you." She smiled at Renee and Benjamin. "Why don't we go to my office and we can talk about what is going to happen?"

Walter interrupted her. "No offense, miss, but I'm not having the surgery. I think we have a misunderstanding here, doc. My wife wanted to come and talk about this . . . prostate thing that I have. I do not want to have surgery. Not now, not ever!"

"No offense taken, sir!" Julie smiled as she responded. "I'm the nurse navigator, Mrs. Humphreys. I help men with prostate cancer navigate what can be a very difficult path. I can certainly explain about your husband's diagnosis if you want to come with me."

Dr. Settler seemed relieved that Julie was taking over. He had a busy clinic and he didn't want to spend a lot of time with the family; that would make his clinic run late, and he had dinner plans with his wife.

Shared decision-making, where the man makes a decision in collaboration with the physician, is important for men with prostate cancer (van Stam et al. 2018). The side effects of the available treatments impact quality of life, so the man's involvement in choosing treatment is important. Being actively involved in this process has been shown to result in satisfaction with treatment and quality of life after treatment (van Stam et al. 2018).

Benjamin stood up, put out his hand to his mother, and helped her out of the chair. Walter didn't have a choice, so he, too, got up out of the chair and followed Julie out of the doctor's office and down the hallway. Julie's office was small with shelves lining one wall. The shelves were filled with books and piles of pamphlets. Julie saw Benjamin looking at the pamphlets.

"I gave Mr. Humphreys some of those pamphlets when I saw him the first time. Did you share those with your family, sir?"

Walter looked guilty; he couldn't remember what he had done with them. But he covered his guilt with a gruff response. "I'd rather hear it from the horse's mouth, but the horse seems to have left us with the stable girl!"

Benjamin and Renee answered at the same time. "Walter!" "Dad!"

They were embarrassed by how rude he was. But Julie just smiled.

"It's okay. In my experience, men often want to talk only to the urologist, but I think I'm a better teacher than Dr. Settler so hopefully you'll trust me even if Mr. Humphreys doesn't!" Julie had a smile on her face when she said this.

Renee glared at her husband and he looked down at his shoes. That was very rude of him, he knew, and shooting the messenger was not a good strategy.

"Sorry Miss Julie," he said softly, "I'm just feeling pressured, that's all. I don't want to be cut . . . you know . . . the surgery. And, well, Renee please forgive me, but you want me to have the surgery . . . and well, this is *me* you're talking about, and I don't want to do that!"

It is not easy to decide about what treatment would be best, especially when there are multiple treatment options. The man and his family members may have different opinions about treatment; being in possession of accurate information about the impact of treatment on quality of life is vital when making a treatment decision.

Julie listened and watched as Walter talked to his wife. She had spent the last five years as a nurse navigator and had witnessed the struggles that men go through in the process of making a decision about treatment.

"How about we go about this as if none of you had been part of any appointments that Mr. Humphreys has been to. That way you will all hear the same information and perhaps this will help you to understand his treatment options."

"Sounds good to me!" Benjamin wanted all the information he could get. When he talked to two of the physicians he played basketball with, he got different answers. One of them said that Walter should have the surgery, no questions asked. The other said that at Walter's age, he should get radiation therapy because the surgery was dangerous for an older man. Neither opinion was helpful to him.

Renee thought that more information was just a waste of time. She wanted him to have the surgery and nothing was going to change her mind. The ladies in her church group had suggested that she leave the decision up to Walter. One of them had a husband going through the same thing, and she was vocal in her encouragement to just let Walter decide. Benjamin wanted to hear more from this Julie woman, and Walter did not seem to be listening to his own wife, so maybe Julie could change his mind.

"I'm going to start at the very beginning with the results of the biopsy." Julie talked for the next twenty-five minutes. She stopped often and asked the family if they had any questions or needed clarification about something she had said. She had a book with diagrams that she showed to them and she even drew on a whiteboard on the wall to explain the various treatments.

Renee found herself growing more and more impressed with the young woman, but she certainly didn't seem to be changing Walter's mind. Her husband sat there with a small smile on his face. Renee wasn't sure what he was smiling at or even why he was smiling. She couldn't help herself and she interrupted Julie. "Walter, why do you look like the cat that's got the cream?"

Walter didn't say anything. In his mind, the things that Julie was describing made the case for him not having the surgery. She had described the pee problems and she even talked about, well, things that should not be talked about in mixed company! He was not pleased with that at all, but Benjamin seemed fascinated; he was even taking notes on his phone as she talked! Walter admitted to himself that he had not heard much about the radiation she was talking about. He had thought that it was either surgery or nothing and this other treatment sounded interesting. Maybe it would get his wife off his back.

"So those are the treatments that you can choose from, Mr. Humphreys. There's the surgery or radiation." Julie was wrapping up her talk. "You don't have to make a decision today and the pamphlets I gave you when I first met you are there to help you as well. I can also see you all again at any time, but based on your biopsy results, you should be making a decision in the next couple of weeks."

Walter sighed, and Renee looked annoyed. Now that he had more information, Walter felt that maybe there was an alternative to the surgery. Renee was confused by what Julie had said; she still wanted him to get the surgery so that she would not have to worry about his cancer coming back. As well, she didn't understand why Walter had to choose his treatment. Isn't that what doctors are for? And Dr. Settler had said that Walter should have surgery! Benjamin thanked the nurse navigator profusely; the information she had provided them was very useful in his mind, way more than what his doctor friends had given him.

Receiving more information about treatment may, in some cases, make the treatment decision more difficult! Having a professional such as a nurse navigator or patient educator involved in the process can be very helpful.

Something that Julie said stuck in Renee's mind. Julie said that she had given Walter pamphlets, but why had he not given them to her? She made a mental note to talk to him about that. Was he hiding something from her? She didn't say anything in front of Benjamin and waited till she and her husband were in the car.

"What pamphlets did that woman talk about? Did she give you something that you have not shared with me?" Her voice was angry even though she didn't want this to turn into a fight. They had many disagreements in their marriage. Walter was old-fashioned in his opinions and thought that the man was the natural leader in the family. Renee did not like this and had told him many times that it was *she* who led, most of the time, at least. Partly, this was because his work often meant he was absent when a problem happened. Her involvement in the church and the charity work that she did with her "sisters" had encouraged in her the confidence she lacked in her earlier years. Their disagreements had lessened since they were both retired, but his cancer was something else entirely, and she was prepared to fight with him for as long as it took for him to get treatment.

"I have the stuff, Renee, don't go getting all mad at me. I think it's all in the trunk of the car, and you can have every last bit of it when we get home. I thought the doctor had told me enough about the surgery that I decided I didn't want treatment. But this Julie person made sense. Maybe I need to think about the radiation."

Walter was as good as his word. He found the pamphlets in the trunk of his car and gave them to his wife. She read them that afternoon and found that they pretty much agreed with what the nurse navigator had told them. Maybe surgery wasn't the right thing for Walter after all. She gave the pile of pamphlets to Benjamin, who looked through them quickly and gave them back to her.

"I checked a whole lot of websites on the internet and I think I've got a good handle on things, Mom. Did you find these any helpful?"

"I did indeed, Benjamin," replied Renee, "They agree with what Julie explained. I've changed my mind. I think your dad should have the radiation."

"Mmm," was Benjamin's response. In his reading on the internet he had found information that made him think that his father should have surgery after all. "Take it out and never have to think about it again" was the message he took away from what he had read. The websites he had found all looked professional and some of them had testimonials from men who had robotic surgery. The photos showed men of all ages, both African American and Caucasian, and this made Benjamin feel comfortable about the advice on the websites in addition to the information they provided. He was puzzled by his mother's change of heart about the surgery.

> There is a lot of information on the internet and not all of it is trustworthy. Websites from established institutions such as the Centers for Disease Control and Prevention (CDC) and the American Cancer Society contain accurate information about a variety of cancers. Websites that promise what sounds like a miracle cure and/or no side effects are usually trying to sell you something and may not come through with what they promise.

"What made you change your mind, Mom?" Benjamin asked.

"Well . . . a couple of things, son. Those pamphlets agreed with the stuff Julie told us. And they were easy to read. I liked the pictures they had in them too. But most of all, I changed my mind after I prayed about this. My sisters in the church said that I should leave it up to your dad to decide. And he is the one with the cancer, and it's his body. Your dad is seventy-six years old; I would feel just terrible if I pushed him into surgery and then something bad happened."

Benjamin thought about this for a moment. He respected his mother and if she had changed her mind, maybe he should too. If he was being honest with himself, some of the testimonials on the websites seemed too good to be true. His physician friend had told him that the side effects of the surgery were not pleasant, and his father had said that he was scared of them too. But the websites didn't mention much about side effects. Perhaps it was time for a family meeting.

That weekend, Benjamin called his parents and asked if he could come over to talk about what they had learned from Julie and what they, or rather, Walter wanted to do next. Walter was tired of all the talking, but Renee took any opportunity to spend time with Benjamin, so he reluctantly agreed. Benjamin was sitting on the balcony of his parents' apartment talking to his father when Renee arrived from church.

"What are you two talking about?" Renee was annoyed that they had not waited for her.

"Oh shush, dear," Walter was smiling at his wife who looked good in her navy suit and white hat with a navy feather. "We're talking about the grandsons, that's all. Did you know that Ben Jr. has started playing golf?"

"Yes, I did know that, and I think it's a fine thing! Now let me get out of these shoes before I suffer any more. Do you boys want something to drink?"

The two men shook their head and watched as Renee kicked off her "Sunday shoes." Why do women torture themselves for the sake of vanity? Walter thought to himself. He glanced at his son and knew he was thinking the same thing. They smiled at each other as they waited for Renee to return. When she appeared and settled herself into a chair with a sigh, Benjamin started to talk.

"Dad, time is passing and I think that you need to be deciding what treatment you're going to have. I think I can speak for Mom in that we are worried about you. It's been months since you found out about the cancer, and it's not going away by itself. When are you going to decide?"

"Settle down, boy!" Walter sounded annoyed. "Who says I haven't decided?"

Renee opened her mouth to speak but Walter gave her one of his looks and she said nothing.

"I talked with that nice girl, Julie, and I am going to see a radiologist next week!" Walter looked pleased with himself.

"A radiologist? Dad, that's a person who takes X-rays! Why are you going to have X-rays?" Benjamin was confused, but the next moment he realized that Walter had the kind of specialist wrong. "Oh, you mean you're going to see a radiation *oncologist*!"

"That's what I said! A radiation . . . what did you say? On-col . . ."

"A radiation *oncologist* is a cancer doctor who uses radiation to treat cancer. Oh, never mind the details . . . when are you going to see him?"

"Next Tuesday at 9 o'clock. Julie made the appointment for me. She's very helpful, that Julie!"

"Well, thank you for telling me!" Renee was now annoyed. "Are you intending to go alone again? You know what Julie said! She said that you should always go with someone to doctor appointments! What did she say that was so cute? Oh yes, four ears are better than two and your two ears don't hear so well these days!"

"So, is this for a second opinion, or are you seriously considering radiation?" Benjamin was puzzled; he thought his father was opposed to any treatment at all.

"I'll decide after I've seen the radiation doctor. Julie said that I really should have treatment and so far, she's making good sense. She even asked me if I wanted her to go with me to the appointment, and I said yes."

Renee and Benjamin looked at each other; this was a real turnaround for Walter, and it seemed as if Julie was the one who had influenced the change.

Seeking a second opinion is quite common for men newly diagnosed with prostate cancer. They may want more information about their cancer or to find the "best" doctor to treat them (Radhakrishnan et al. 2017). However, it may cause more confusion, as most specialists have a good rationale for why their treatment is the best.

Renee went with Walter to the appointment the following week; but Benjamin could not get off work. Julie was waiting for them in the lobby of the building where the doctor's office was located.

"Hello again!" she greeted them and ushered their way to the elevator. As they were going up to the sixth floor, Julie peppered Walter with questions and, to Renee's amazement, he didn't seem bothered by what felt like a game of twenty questions. He answered her and was his charming best, something that Renee had missed over the past few months since his diagnosis. She had felt disconnected from him and any conversation now felt like there was a dark cloud in the room.

They waited just a few minutes before being invited into the doctor's office. To Walter's surprise, the radiation oncologist was a woman. He was not used to female health care providers, and Renee worried that this would be a challenge for him.

"Hello Mr. Humphreys and Mrs. Humphreys. I'm Dr. Patel." The doctor appeared to be in her early fifties and was short, with a broad smile. "Hello Julie! Nice to see you too!"

She gestured to a pair of chairs on the other side of her desk. She immediately realized that Julie did not have anywhere to sit; she picked up her phone and asked someone to bring another chair to her office. Within minutes they were all seated, and the radiation oncologist started to speak.

"Mr. Humphreys, I have the results of your biopsy right here on my computer," she turned the monitor so that he could see what she was referring to. "The good news is that your cancer is very treatable. We have a number of treatments using radiation that are all effective. I know that Julie does a really good job of explaining things to patients, so if you have some questions about radiation, I will try to answer them to the best of my ability."

Renee looked at her husband; Dr. Patel's approach was so different from the other doctor they had seen. Walter seemed a little shocked that he was being encouraged to ask questions. He looked at Julie, who smiled at him and nodded her head slightly.

"Well, doc . . ." Walter began; he did not look comfortable and Renee reached over and patted his knee. "In the beginning I didn't want to have anything done to me at all. I've never been in the hospital before, and I've always been healthy. I had to be, for my work, you know. But the other doctor I saw, well, he wanted to do the surgery and that scared me, so I thought I'd do nothing. But my wife and my son, they wanted me to do the surgery. Then I met Julie here, and she changed my mind. I want to do something for my cancer, but I'm not sure what. Julie said that I could choose, but I know nothing about this! I'm not a doctor."

Walter sighed and looked at Dr. Patel.

"You sound like a lot of my patients, Mr. Humphreys. We do ask men to choose their treatment, because every treatment has side effects that impact your quality of life. We don't know you and your values, and so it would not be fair for us to tell you what treatment to have. Of course, there are some men who cannot have surgery for any number of reasons and so they have to have radiation, and vice versa. And some men don't need treatment immediately and we can monitor them carefully over time. But the vast majority of men, like you, do have a choice. May I ask Mrs. Humphreys what she thinks?

Renee looked surprised that someone was asking her opinion. "Well, doctor . . . I want the best for my husband. I've prayed about this a lot. I don't know why this happened to him. He's a good man. A good father and grandfather. My sisters at church have told me that *he* needs to decide about treatment. But I want him to have the surgery, to take it out, and then it's over. I don't really understand about this radiation, but if you can explain it to me, then maybe I will know more."

Renee was surprised that she had talked so much. She looked at Walter, expecting him to be angry, but instead he was smiling at her. Now it was his turn to pat her on the knee.

It is important that the man understand *why* he is being asked to participate in shared decision-making and he needs to have enough information to make an informed choice. Not infrequently, important information about side effects, especially sexual side effects, is not provided and, as a result, the man experiences treatment regret months or years afterward. (Wagland et al. 2019)

"So . . . let me explain . . ." Dr. Patel looked from one to the other and in simple terms, told them how radiation worked. She described the side effects that were possible and even probable and told them how long they may last and what could be done to lessen them. She paused often as she talked to them and asked if either of them had any questions. A lot of what she said they knew already, especially about the side effects, because Julie had told them about that. When she was done, she sat back in her chair with a small smile on her face.

"That was a lot of information, and I hope I haven't confused you."

Walter and Renee both responded at the same time. "No, that was good!" They laughed at what they had just done. Renee felt that she and her husband were on the same page for the first time in a very long time.

Dr. Patel was not finished. "Mr. Humphreys, you do not need to make a decision right here and now. Go home and talk to your wife and anyone else who is important to you. But remember, this is *your* decision to make, and you should make it with consideration of your values. I am here if you have any other questions or if you want another appointment with me. And Julie is a good resource for you too. Take some time deciding what you want to do, but don't take too much time. Not making a decision will only delay your return to a normal life for you and your family."

Renee felt a weight lift off her shoulders. If radiation is what Walter decided, then it was a good decision. She had faith in this doctor and her life depended on her faith. For the first time, she felt at peace with the whole situation. It was a good feeling.

CONCLUSION

It is not easy to make a treatment decision, and many men with prostate cancer don't know that they have a choice as to what treatment they have. If they are not fully informed about their choices, they may accept the recommendation of the first and only provider they see. Accessing accurate and unbiased information is an important first step. Family members should receive the same information so that they can be supportive in the decision-making process and not pressure the man to do what they think is the right decision.

Reflective Questions

After reading this chapter:

- How might you persuade your partner/spouse to have treatment without causing conflict?
- What do you think is the role of family members in encouraging your partner/spouse to have treatment?
- How do you find resources to help you and your partner/spouse understand the facts about prostate cancer and its treatments?

REFERENCES

Airhihenbuwa, C. O., and L. Liburd. 2006. "Eliminating health disparities in the African American population: The interface of culture, gender, and power." *Health Education & Behavior* 33 (4): 488–501. doi: 10.1177/1090198106287731.

Radhakrishnan, A., D. Grande, N. Mitra, J. Bekelman, C. Stillson, and C. E. Pollack. 2017. "Second opinions from urologists for prostate cancer: Who gets them, why, and their link to treatment." *Cancer* 123 (6): 1027–34. doi: 10.1002/cncr.30412.

Siegel, R., K. Miller, A. Jemal. 2020. "Cancer Statistics, 2020." *CA: Cancer Journal for Clinicians* 70 (1): 7–30. doi: 10.3322/caac.21590.

van Stam, M. A., A. H. Pieterse, H. G. van der Poel, J. Bosch, C. Tillier, S. Horenblas, and N. K. Aaronson. 2018. "Shared decision making in prostate cancer care-encouraging every patient to be actively involved in decision making or ensuring the patient preferred level of involvement?" *Journal of Urology* 200 (3): 582–89. doi: 10.1016/j.juro.2018.02.3091.

Vapiwala, N., D. Miller, B. Laventure, K. Woodhouse, S. Kelly, J. Avelis, C. Baffic, R. Goldston, and K. Glanz. 2021. "Stigma, beliefs and perceptions regarding prostate cancer among Black and Latino men and women." *BMC Public Health* 21 (1): 758. doi: 10.1186/s12889-021-10793-x.

Wagland, R., J. Nayoan, L. Matheson, C. Rivas, J. Brett, A. Downing, S. Wilding, H. Butcher, A. Gavin, A. W. Glaser, and E. Watson. 2019. "'Very difficult for an ordinary guy': Factors influencing the quality of treatment decision-making amongst men diagnosed with localised and locally advanced prostate cancer: Findings from a UK-wide mixed methods study." *Patient Education and Counselling* 102 (4): 797–803. doi: 10.1016/j.pec.2018.12.004.

Williams, D. R., and T. D. Rucker. 2000. "Understanding and addressing racial disparities in health care." *Health Care Financing Review* 21 (4): 75–90.

Chapter Four

Active Surveillance

Delaying Treatment

The couple in this chapter is dealing with a treatment option, active surveillance, that has been recommended, but the man's spouse and their adult children are opposed to this treatment. The couple's relationship is strained by his decision and both suffer because of misunderstandings and lack of knowledge.

Brian and Rosemary Porter have been married for almost forty years. Brian is a college professor who teaches English to graduate students; he had planned to retire soon, but the downturn in the stock market has caused him some uncertainly about this. Rosemary is the same age as her husband, sixty-two, and she is a retired accountant. They have two grown children; Jude is thirty-four years old and the CEO of a tech start-up. Michelle is thirty-two and a doctoral student studying twentieth-century American literature. Both young adults live near their parents, and the family is close.

Brian's father died ten years ago at the age of seventy-seven from an aggressive prostate cancer. Ever since his father's death, Brian has had a PSA test every year. And every year he grows anxious in the days leading up to having the test and then waiting the twenty-four hours for the results. Despite almost ten years of the results being normal, he still can't control his anxiety. His primary care provider at the college health service, Brenda, is an experienced primary care nurse practitioner. Over the years she has learned that it is useless to try and make suggestions to alleviate his anxiety; he just needs to get through the days until he receives the result and then he calms down instantly. But this year his PSA was slightly elevated.

Brenda referred him to a urologist, and he had a biopsy a week later. He learned the results two weeks after that, when the urologist called him on his cell phone; he had low-risk prostate cancer that was of low volume. At least that was what he thought he heard. Despite his belief that, because his father had prostate cancer, he would eventually be diagnosed too, he was shocked. The first person he called was his brother-in-law Mitch, who was married to his sister. He and Mitch were not that close, but Mitch was the only medical person in the extended family. Mitch was an anesthesiologist and was always prepared to give his opinion on any health-related issue, even if it was not something he knew a lot about.

> While it is common and convenient to ask a family member who is a medical professional for advice about cancer, it is important to remember that the field of medicine or nursing is very broad and complex. Asking a family member for advice also puts pressure on them to comment, and this may make them uncomfortable because they want to help and feel unable to refuse.

The first question Brian asked Mitch was "Is what happened to my dad going to happen to me?"

Mitch didn't know much about the role that family history played in the development or prognosis of prostate cancer. "I really don't know, Brian. Have you seen a urologist? What about your family physician? What did he say?"

"You're the first person I called," Brian replied. "I haven't even told Rosemary yet! I thought you might know what this means. I saw a urologist who did the biopsy, but he just called me on the phone with the results. I haven't seen my nurse practitioner yet. I guess I should call her to make an appointment."

Mitch was surprised with what he heard. He thought that the urologist would have made a follow-up appointment to discuss treatment and he wondered why a cancer diagnosis was told to the patient on the phone. "Yeah, you need to see the urologist for sure. And I guess your nurse practitioner might be able to explain this as well. I didn't know you saw a nurse."

"I've been seeing Brenda for years. She's at the college health clinic and she's amazing. Takes as much time as I need, and she explains everything so well." Brian was irritated with his brother-in-law's attitude. He liked Brenda and he trusted her, and he hoped that she would know what to do now that the inevitable, in his opinion, had happened. But he needed to talk to his wife and then his kids. This was not going to be easy.

It was as difficult to tell Rosemary as he anticipated. As much as he believed that he would eventually get the same cancer as his father, Rosemary had always hoped that this was not his destiny. She was the one who tried to keep him calm when he waited for the results of his PSA tests, and she had tried to reassure him that everything would be okay after he had his biopsy. After he said the words—"I have prostate cancer"—they hugged each other for a long time. Rosemary tried to not cry; she didn't want to upset Brian, but still the tears rolled down her cheeks.

Brian broke their embrace. He gently wiped the tears from her face and tried to smile. "I made an appointment to see Brenda tomorrow to talk about what this means. The urologist said something about 'low risk' but honestly, I didn't hear much after he told me I had cancer."

"Can I come with you to that appointment?" Rosemary was scared to ask; he was private about some things and health was top of that list.

"I guess you should—*we* should—both hear the same thing." Brian sounded tentative. Rosemary hugged him again.

Many people do not hear much after they hear the words "you have cancer" (Friis et al. 2003). The diagnosis itself is experienced as something traumatic to begin with, followed by a period when they "take on" the challenge of having cancer. This is often followed by "taking control" of the disease and treatment. (McCaughan and McKenna 2007)

Brian and Rosemary were early for his appointment with the nurse practitioner. She did not keep them waiting and greeted them where they sat in the waiting room.

"Let's go to my office. It's a bit messy but it's better than an examination room."

Brian did not think her office was messy at all. His office in the English Department a few buildings over was much less tidy; there were piles of books on every horizontal surface, and some on the floor. His colleagues at the college had stopped remarking about what they saw as chaos. There were two mismatched chairs and a small desk with a laptop in Brenda's office; it was obvious that she didn't use the office all that much. Brian and Rosemary sat down on the chairs, one of which had one leg a little shorter than the other three, so it wobbled.

"Sorry about that, folks. The college doesn't give really have money for these things. But you must know about that, Brian, right?"

Brian nodded. Budgets were always tight at the college, and it was clear that the health services were as neglected as the rest of the departments.

Rosemary was not impressed by what she saw. Her first thought was concern that the care her husband received at the clinic was as poor as the office where they now sat. She looked over at Brian, who seemed unconcerned. He had been coming to this clinic ever since he first starting teaching at the college and he had never commented on the shabbiness of the place.

"Let me just pull up the results of your biopsy, Brian. I requested them from the urologist, and they should have been scanned in by now. Yes, here they are." Brenda had her back to the couple at first, but she turned around to face them. "I'm going to go through the results with you, but please interrupt me and ask any questions. From what I can see, the pathology report says that three of the twelve samples showed some cancer and the grade of the cancer is reported as low risk. Does that make sense to you both?"

Brian grunted; Rosemary was not sure what that meant but she certainly didn't understand anything about this. The nurse practitioner continued to explain, but Rosemary tuned out her voice. All she could think about was losing her husband of so many years. She had retired just a couple of months before, and Brian was going to follow her, but he was not sure about his pension and their investments; they were supposed to travel and do all the things they had put off because of work. And now this . . .

"Rose, honey? Are you listening?" Brian's voice interrupted her thoughts. "I think this is good news, isn't it?" He looked at Brenda and then back at his wife.

"I'm sorry, I drifted off there for a minute," Rosemary was embarrassed. "What were you saying?"

Brian sighed. Brenda had gone over his results and he was buoyed by the explanation she had provided. But Rosemary had not listened to any of it! He was embarrassed and annoyed.

"Do you want Brenda to go over everything again?" His voice reflected his frustration.

"I don't want to waste any more time. You must be very busy." Rosemary stood up to leave.

"It's not a problem, Mrs. Porter." the nurse practitioner tried to help what had now become uncomfortable. "I have some reading material for you as well as information about support groups for both of you."

"That'll be helpful, thank you." Brian was not sure what else to say. He got up reluctantly and followed his wife out of the office. He was angry now but managed to keep quiet until they reached his car.

"Seriously Rosemary! Do you even realize how rude you were? I'm mortified by your behavior!"

To his surprise, his wife burst into tears. He had expected her to argue with him or at least justify her behavior but, instead, she was sobbing. "It's so scary! Why is this happening to us?"

Rosemary was usually the calm one in their relationship, but she was anything but that now. Brian wanted to remind her that it was happening to *him* but telling her that was not going to help.

"Brenda suggested that I go and see the urologist again. She said that they often just watch things in cases like mine and she wanted me to hear about my treatment options from a specialist. She's going to ask his office to see me sooner rather than later."

His wife nodded, got into the car, and remained silent on the trip home.

Later that day, Brian received a call from the urologist's office with an appointment for the end of the week. He knocked on the bedroom door where Rosemary had been since they got home. He was confused by her behavior; she seemed more upset than he was, and he was the person with cancer! He hoped she would pull herself together and soon!

They went to see the urologist together. Rosemary had brought a notebook with her and she occupied herself while they were waiting by writing down questions in her neat handwriting. Brian was pleased about this; he didn't know what to ask, despite having read the material that Brenda had given him.

The urologist shook Brian's hand and then introduced himself to Rosemary. Dr. Sheridan loosened his tie as he sat down. He seemed rather young to Rosemary, but he had an air of confidence and seemed friendly. He went over Brian's biopsy results, and this time she listened intently.

"Mr. Porter . . . may I call you Brian? Okay, so in a nutshell you have low-risk, low-volume disease. This is good news, and I think we should just watch this. That way we can delay surgery for as long as possible. Any questions?"

Rosemary looked up from her notebook where she had been writing down his every word. "Yes, I have some questions, if I may . . ." She glanced at Brian, who nodded at her to go ahead. His mind was whirling with questions of his own, but he was happy to let her take the lead. "My husband's father died of prostate cancer, so I don't understand why you are suggesting that we, that he, doesn't do anything about his cancer!" Her voice had risen an octave or two and Brian grimaced. He didn't want her to get angry or cry. That would not be helpful.

"Ah . . . this is a common question, Mrs. Porter. I am not suggesting that we do nothing. What I am proposing is something called active surveillance. We now recognize that for years we have overtreated low-risk prostate cancer and, to prevent this, we now actively monitor the man's cancer, hence the term active surveillance. Let me explain . . ."

The intent of the active surveillance is to prevent the side effects of the other treatments. As you will read in the following chapters, the side effects of surgery and radiation therapy impact on urinary, bowel, and sexual functions, all of which negatively affect the man's quality of life. (Venderbos et al. 2017)

"I don't understand," Rosemary was getting more upset, "My husband's father didn't get treatment either, and he died of his cancer!"

Dr. Sheridan took a deep breath and responded to her. "The important thing to remember here is that your father-in-law's prostate cancer is not your husband's cancer. A family history is an indication for screening for prostate cancer with regular PSA tests, but one person's outcome does not predict the outcome for his family member. Does that make sense to you?"

"Not really, Dr. Sheridan. Can you clarify that please? I'm sorry to be asking so many questions but, well, I don't want to have to see my husband go through what his father did! It was awful." Rosemary struggled to keep her voice under control and she was close to tears.

Some studies suggest that a family history of prostate cancer increases the risk of being diagnosed with the same cancer (Barber et al. 2018), others suggest that a family history does not increase the risk of having a more aggressive form of the disease or of the disease progressing. (Telang et al. 2017)

Rosemary interrupted the doctor. "But that's what they did with Brian's dad and he died! They watched and they waited—for him to die!"

Brian had been silent through all of this. He wanted to ask the same questions as his wife, but she was much braver than him in the moment.

"Ah, yes, this is a common misperception about active surveillance and what we call "watchful waiting,'" responded Dr. Sheridan. His voice showed no sign of frustration as he continued to explain. "We used to do something called watchful waiting years ago. Watchful waiting meant that the man was not treated until he experienced symptoms from the cancer. It was mostly used in elderly patients who were not expected to live for a long time. I know this sounds strange, but the risks of surgery are significant for an elderly man."

"I don't think my dad was given a choice," Brian said softly. "He died when he was seventy-seven, and I think he was diagnosed a couple of years before that. I don't remember any details of what happened back then. He was a very private man, my dad, and he didn't talk about things, not until near the end. That's when I started with the PSA tests."

"You did the right thing to start early PSA screening." Dr. Sheridan continued, "Would you like to hear more about what we do with active surveillance? I do think this is the right course for you at this time, but you can choose to have surgery or even radiation if that would make you more comfortable."

Rosemary turned to her husband. "Is this what you want to do? I'm not sure but it's your call."

"Let's just listen to what the doctor has to say. I want to hear all my options and if he thinks this is the way to go."

"I want to emphasize that what I am proposing is active management of your prostate cancer. We will do regular PSA tests as well as digital rectal examinations. I want you to have a baseline MRI as well, and I will do another biopsy in a year. Hopefully there will not be any progression, and we will continue the monitoring for as long as you feel comfortable. At any time, you can change your mind and opt for surgery."

Brian was nodding his head as the urologist spoke. The side effects of surgery had not sounded like something he wanted to experience, and if this active monitoring worked, even in the short term, he was certainly interested.

The American Urological Association recommends PSA tests every three months for the first year of surveillance, then every three to six months during and after the second year (https://www.auanet.org/guidelines/guidelines/prostate-cancer-clinically-localized-guideline#x6906). Repeating the biopsy six months to one year after initial diagnosis and then every three to five years is recommended. (Chen et al. 2016)

Rosemary looked at Brian; he was smiling and nodding, and her heart sunk. Had they heard the same thing from the urologist? She was not sure about this way of proceeding at all, and she was surprised that the doctor had not suggested surgery. That would take care of the cancer, and he would be done with treatment.

"Dr. Sheridan, if I may?" Rosemary wanted to ask her questions before Brian agreed to this. "Isn't this just delaying the inevitable? I mean, if he lands up having surgery in a year or two, why do this?"

"A lot of people ask me that exact question, Mrs. Porter, and I prefer to think that we are *deferring* treatment for as long as possible. In this way, your husband doesn't suffer the side effects of surgery and his quality of life remains the same as it is now."

"But what if the cancer comes back?"

"That is why we do the PSA tests very regularly and another biopsy within a year." Dr. Sheridan was patient with Rosemary; he was used to this kind of response, often from family members and not the man with prostate cancer.

"And what are the side effects of just watching the cancer?" Rosemary was not giving up on her argument against this.

"Other than some men experiencing anxiety before routine monitoring, you know, while they wait for the results of the blood test or biopsy, there aren't any," replied Dr. Sheridan with confidence. "That's the whole point of doing this! The man doesn't have any other side effects!"

At this point, Brian was getting tired of Rosemary's questions. He stood up and put out his hand to shake the doctor's hand. "Okay, that's it then. I've made my decision and I am going to do this. What do I need to do now, Doctor?"

"My receptionist will schedule another appointment for us in the coming months. You'll need to have your PSA measured every three months . . . we'll arrange that. Good to meet you, Brian! And don't worry, Mrs. Porter, we'll take good care of your man here!"

"Thank you, Dr. Sheridan. Rose, honey, let's go . . . c'mon now. Let's not waste any more of the doctor's time."

Rosemary got up reluctantly; she had more questions, but her husband was not interested it seemed to her. She was still not convinced about what Brian had decided but was there any point in arguing?

By the time they got home, Rosemary had hatched a plan; she was going to talk to Jude and Michelle, and they would persuade their dad to have surgery. Brian had not told them about his diagnosis yet, but she felt she had to talk to them. After dropping her off at home, Brian went straight to his office at the college. All the time he had spent with appointments over the last while had made him behind on working on a new curriculum for his postgraduate seminar for the next semester and he needed to get that done.

While he was at work, Rosemary texted her two children and asked them to meet her at a nearby coffee shop. Michelle was at home working on something for one of her courses at university and, luckily, Jude could get away from his work for an hour. When they all had their drinks, they sat outside the coffee shop at a small table, some distance away from other people. She felt guilty telling them about Brian's cancer before he had, but someone had to do something about the mistake he was making, and *she* was that someone.

She quickly told them what had happened over the past weeks. She had to look at her notes from the appointment with the urologist and as she talked, she realized that she was not presenting a balanced recounting of what had been said, but she was desperate to get Jude and Michelle onside. It didn't take much to persuade them; both young adults readily agreed to help her change their father's mind and have surgery. The conversation then moved to figuring out a strategy to talk to him. That took a little longer; Michelle did not want them to seem to be ganging up on him, but Jude told her that desperate times call for desperate measures and they had to do whatever they could to persuade him.

It is not unusual for family members to want the man to have surgery, as they believe that this will cure the cancer (Brooks et al. 2018). Their beliefs about the cancer and its treatment may be based on the experience of other people that they know or have heard about, despite everyone's cancer and response to treatment being unique.

That weekend, Jude and Michelle arrived just in time for Sunday lunch. Brian was caught off guard but then realized that his wife had prepared food for four and not just the two of them. What was this about? He had planned to talk to them about his diagnosis, but he was so busy at work that he had delayed it. They had just filled their plates with food when Michelle took the lead in questioning him.

"Dad, how could you keep this from us? You have *cancer* and you didn't tell us! What is wrong with you?"

Brian glared at his wife. What right did she have to tell them? Before he could say anything, Jude put in his two cents' worth.

"Dad, have you thought this through? I agree with Mom. You have made a rash decision to not have surgery and I, we, want you to reconsider!"

Brian put down his fork, pushed his chair away from the table, and stood up. "Rosemary? Really, you told them? This was not yours to tell! How could you?" He left the dining room, stormed up the stairs, and slammed the bedroom door closed.

His family sat in silence, their eyes on their plates.

Jude broke the quiet. "That didn't go well . . . what do we do now?"

Michelle got up from the table. She had tears in her eyes as she ran from the room.

"Let her go, Jude," Rosemary told her son. "She'll be back."

But Michelle did not come back, at least not for a while. She went up the stairs and knocked quietly on the door to her parents' bedroom. "Dad, it's me. Can I come in? Please?"

There was silence for a while and as she was about to knock again, the door opened and Brian was standing there, his face red and an agitated look in his eyes. "If you've come to persuade me, it's no use. I'm hurt and angry, and I don't want to talk about what happened just now!"

"I'm so sorry, Dad," Michelle was crying. "I don't know why it happened this way. I was just hurt because you didn't tell us about what had happened and then Jude said what he said and that is not the way I thought it would go!"

Brian hated it when his daughter cried; it had been this way since she was a little girl. "It's okay, Michie," he said, using his pet name for her. "Don't cry, please, stop crying. I'm mostly angry at your mother for talking to you before I had a chance to. We'll sort that out later, but let me tell you why I decided to do what I'm doing."

Brian explained everything to his daughter. He told her the whole story, from his visit to Brenda to the appointment with the urologist. He told her about the side effects of both surgery and radiation, leaving out the sexual problems, of course. He described what active surveillance meant. Michelle listened without saying a word until he finished.

"Hmm, that's not what Mom told us. She said that if you had the surgery then everything would be okay. She didn't talk about side effects and they sound horrible! Why didn't she tell us what you just told me?"

"Your Mom thinks that I should have the surgery, she's convinced of it. But this is my body and no matter what she says, I'm doing this active surveillance and that's that. Now let's go back downstairs and I'll put an end to this revolution that you've cooked up!"

They joined Rosemary and Jude at the table. Brian was much calmer now and he explained to Jude why he had made the decision to avoid surgery or any other treatment for now. He tried to persuade Rosemary and Jude that active surveillance was safe, and that careful monitoring would pick up any changes in his cancer that could then be acted on with either surgery or radiation. Jude stared at his mother when Brian described the side effects of the surgery. Why did she not tell them about this part? She had made it seem so clear: surgery would cure the cancer and that would be the end of it. What his father described was certainly different. Rosemary looked embarrassed as her husband talked to their children. She knew that what she had done was wrong, and she also knew that she had to apologize to them but especially to Brian.

It had taken a lot of persuading but, as time went by, Michelle and Jude seemed less focused on his health and things went back to normal. His PSA did not go up and he was pleased with his decision. Michelle was engrossed in her studies and preparing for her research and Jude was focused on his start-up that seemed to be doing well. After an initial period of a couple of weeks, within which Rosemary remained mad at him, things settled down between them. Rosemary stopped badgering him and seemed to accept his decision. Brian was busy with teaching his assigned courses. The revisions he had made to the graduate seminar were working well and he had two new doctoral students to supervise.

The months went by, and one day as he was leaving the college, he received a phone call from Dr. Sheridan's office; it had been almost a year since his first biopsy, and it was time for the next one. Since Rosemary had stopped nagging him about "doing nothing" as she called it, they hardly talked about his cancer. Brian was a little surprised that she let the topic go; she seemed to have calmed down and he was grateful for that.

For the first time, Brian felt a slight tingle of apprehension. He considered not telling his family about the biopsy appointment but thought better of it. The last time he hid information from them it did not go well.

Most people will experience some anxiety before having a test that monitors whether their cancer has progressed. There is no right or wrong way to cope and it may be difficult for the man to change his "natural" coping style although the more negative ways of coping may result in distress.

Later that evening, Brian received a call from his brother-in-law. The timing was interesting, Brian thought to himself.

"Hey buddy," Mitch always talked too loudly, and Brian had to hold the phone away from his ear. "So I talked to one of the urologists who operates at my hospital. He had some interesting things to say. Do you want to hear them?"

Brian's immediate response was irritation that Mitch had talked about him to another doctor. But perhaps this other urologist had information that might be useful to him. "Sure, go ahead, Mitch."

"So this was a surprise to me too. The guy I talked to, well he said that this monitoring thing is the way to go and that he suggests it to a lot of his patients. Who knew?"

Brian smiled at this. He appreciated Mitch telling him this, especially since what he said reinforced his decision.

Mitch continued. "He also said that most men on this don't go on to develop metastatic cancer, you know, spread of the cancer."

"I know what that means, Mitch," Brian couldn't help himself from pointing out to his brother-in-law that he understood some of this cancer language. "But thanks. This confirms what my doctor said, and my nurse practitioner too!"

There has been a significant increase in urologists recommending active surveillance for their patients with low-risk prostate cancer over the past decade and this approach appears to be safe (Mahal et al. 2019). Even if the man eventually decides to have surgery, or if there is disease progression, the outcomes from surgery are as good as they are for men who have immediate surgery (Ahmad et al. 2020).

He told Rosemary about the upcoming biopsy one week before his appointment. He could see the anxiety in her eyes as soon as she heard. She wanted to tell Jude and Michelle immediately, but he asked her to wait a couple of days. What was the use in causing them to worry? But he realized that maybe Rosemary needed their support and so he sent them a text telling them the date of his biopsy. Michelle called him immediately; she had a lot of questions about the procedure and when he would receive the results.

"See what has happened?" he said to Rosemary. "What good did telling her do?"

Rosemary didn't answer him. She was trying hard to hide her anxiety from him and she knew that she should not talk about how worried she was. The time seemed to drag by until it was the day of the procedure. To Rosemary, Brian seemed unconcerned. He had taken the antibiotics that Dr. Sheridan prescribed and was up, dressed, and ready to go almost an hour before his early-morning appointment. Rosemary drove him there and decided to wait in the car rather than in the doctor's waiting room. She had a book to read but spent most of the time staring out the window.

Brian had to knock on the passenger-side window to get her to unlock the door. He seemed in a good mood and asked her to drop him off at the college.

"Are you sure? Don't you want to come home and rest?" Rosemary sounded worried, but Brian said he was fine and would rather be occupied at work than be treated as an invalid, which he wasn't.

"I'm fine, really, I am. The biopsy was not big deal, and if I feel bad, I'll call you to pick me up. Is that okay with you?"

Rosemary nodded. Why was he being so brave in the face of something that could be life-changing? She was once again nervous about this active surveillance treatment he had chosen. How could he be so calm? As she drove back home after dropping him off, she thought about the past year. For a while she was consumed with worry about her husband, but as time went by and he seemed the same person that he had always been, her worry decreased. His PSA tests had remained almost the same as before but now they had to wait for the biopsy results. Her brother-in-law Mitch had explained that the biopsy results were more important than the blood tests, and now that Brian had the second biopsy, her anxiety was overwhelming.

By the time Brian called her to pick him up from the college, she was a mess. She had not been able to stop playing a stream of negative scenarios in her head. She imagined them finding out that the cancer had spread and there was nothing that could be done to stop it; that was the worst of her imaginary outcomes. She prepared herself for how she would react if he was sick and if she would be able to care for him when the end came. Another scenario she conjured up was seeing Brian in the hospital after surgery, pain all over his face, as Dr. Sheridan explained to them that he could not remove all the cancer.

She drove to the college with tears pouring down her face. When Brian opened the door of the car, he was shocked at her appearance. Her mascara was smeared down her cheeks and her face puffy.

"What has happened? Are the kids okay? What is it? What's wrong?"

"They're fine," Rosemary's voice was strained, "It's me. I'm so scared. I don't want to lose you!"

"What? How are you going to lose me? What's this about?"

Brian was confused by her outburst. He didn't want to her to drive when she was upset, so he suggested that she move into the passenger seat and he would drive. They were silent on the short drive home other than the occasional sniff from Rosemary. Brian put on the kettle and made himself some tea while his wife watched him closely.

"Are you sure you don't want something to drink? You look like you need a scotch?" His attempt at humor fell flat. With a sigh, he sat down at the kitchen table. "Go on . . . what are you thinking? Why were you so upset?"

Rosemary took a deep breath and told him what she had been imagining. Brian tried to keep a neutral expression on his face, but it was not easy. He was shocked and concerned about how worried she was. He had no idea that she had been thinking such negative thoughts about his cancer.

"I thought you were okay with me doing this surveillance thing. I really thought we were on the same page about this."

"Well, I guess I'm not really! I don't like the idea of you not doing anything about the cancer! What if it spreads? What if I lose you?"

Rosemary was crying again, and he hated it when she cried. It made him feel helpless and he often got angry when this happened.

The anxiety experienced by the spouse/partner of the man with prostate cancer impacts the man himself (Chien et al. 2019). The mental health of a man's spouse is impacted negatively by his diagnosis of prostate cancer (Hyde et al. 2018). Support groups for partners that allow for expression of emotions and social support may help to alleviate distress. (Carlson et al. 2017)

Brian stood up from the table, his tea untouched. "Rose, I just can't handle it when you get like this! It's *me* who's had the biopsy! It's *me* who's dealing with you and Michelle and the pressure you put on *me* to calm you all down! I need some space right now."

"Wait! Brian, don't go!" Rosemary tried to stop her tears, but it was useless. The sight of him walking away made her cry even harder. She stayed at the table, her gaze focused on the mug of tea he had left behind.

He returned ten minutes later by which time the tears had dried on her cheeks and she was breathing normally again. He sat down, pushed away the mug of now lukewarm tea, and put his arm around her shoulders. She sighed and let her head drop onto his chest.

"I'm sorry . . ."—they both spoke at the same time, then laughed softly at themselves.

"Let me go first, please," Rosemary looked at him, her eyes meeting his. "I'm just worried, that's all. I respect your choice, but I'm still scared. Maybe I need to get some help to deal with this."

"That's exactly what I was going to suggest. I can't help you control your worry, but maybe a professional can. I'm going to ask Brenda if she knows where we can get some help for you. Is that okay?"

Rosemary nodded. It was hard for her to accept help, but she knew that she needed it. She could not go on like this, and Brian had not received the results of this second biopsy yet.

Brian threw the now cold tea into the sink and called Brenda; she agreed to see the two of them later that week. At least they had a plan, thought Brian. Now they had to wait.

CONCLUSION

Active surveillance of prostate cancer is increasingly recommended for men with low-risk disease. This does not mean that the man will never have treatment; the man can decide to have surgery or radiation at any time. The careful monitoring of the cancer means that any changes suggestive of progression of the cancer will result in treatment with surgery or radiation. But the thought of the man deferring immediate treatment can be difficult for family members.

Reflective Questions

After reading this chapter:

- What are some concerns you might have in asking a medical professional with little to no expertise about prostate cancer treatment?
- What strategies could be used to help family members understand why a man might choose active surveillance as a treatment option?
- What can the partner of a man on active surveillance do to control their anxiety?

REFERENCES

Ahmad, A. E., P. O. Richard, R. Leão, M. Hajiha, L. J. Martin, M. Komisarenko, R. Grewal, H. Goldberg, S. Salem, K. Jain, A. Oliaei, I. Horyn, N. Timilshina, A. Zlotta, R. Hamilton, G. Kulkarni, N. Fleshner, S. M. H. Alibhaic, and A. Finelli. 2020. "Does time spent on active surveillance adversely affect the pathological and oncologic outcomes in patients undergoing delayed radical prostatectomy?" *Journal of Urology* 204 (3): 476–82. doi: 10.1097/ju.0000000000001070.

Barber, L., T. Gerke, S. C. Markt, S. F. Peisch, K. M. Wilson, T. Ahearn, E. Giovannucci, G. Parmigiani, and L. A. Mucci. 2018. "Family history of breast or prostate cancer and prostate cancer risk." *Clinical Cancer Research* 24 (23): 5910–17. doi: 10.1158/1078-0432.ccr-18-0370.

Brooks, J. V., S. D. Ellis, E. Morrow, K. S. Kimminau, and J. B. Thrasher. 2018. "Patient Factors that influence how physicians discuss active surveillance with low-risk prostate cancer patients: A qualitative study." *American Journal of Men's Health* 12 (5): 1719–27. doi: 10.1177/1557988318785741.

Carlson, L. E., C. R. Rouleau, M. Speca, J. Robinson, and B. D. Bultz. 2017. "Brief supportive-expressive group therapy for partners of men with early stage prostate cancer: lessons learned from a negative randomized controlled trial." *Support Care Cancer* 25 (4): 1035–1041. doi: 10.1007/s00520-016 -3551-1.

Chen, R. C., R. B. Rumble, D. A. Loblaw, A. Finelli, B. Ehdaie, M. R. Cooperberg, S. C. Morgan, S. Tyldesley, J. J. Haluschak, W. Tan, S. Justman, and S. Jain. 2016. "Active surveillance for the management of localized prostate cancer (Cancer Care Ontario Guideline): American Society of Clinical Oncology clinical practice guideline endorsement." *Journal of Clinical Oncology* 34 (18): 2182–90. doi: 10.1200/jco.2015.65.7759.

Chien, C. H., C. K. Chuang, K. L. Liu, S. T. Pang, C. T. Wu, and Y. H. Chang. 2019. "Prostate cancer-specific anxiety and the resulting health-related quality of life in couples." *Journal of Advanced Nursing* 75 (1): 63–74. doi: 10.1111/jan.13828.

Friis, L. S., B. Elverdam, and K. G. Schmidt. 2003. "The patient's perspective." *Supportive Care in Cancer* 11 (3): 162–70. doi: 10.1007/s00520-002-0424 -6.

Hyde, M. K., M. Legg, S. Occhipinti, S. J. Lepore, A. Ugalde, L. Zajdlewicz, K. Laurie, J. Dunn, and S. K. Chambers. 2018. "Predictors of long-term distress in female partners of men diagnosed with prostate cancer." *Psychooncology* 27 (3): 946–54. doi: 10.1002/pon.4617.

Mahal, A. R., S. Butler, I. Franco, V. Muralidhar, D. Larios, L. R. G. Pike, S. G. Zhao, N. N. Sanford, R. T. Dess, F. Y. Feng, A. V. D'Amico, D. E. Spratt, J. B. Yu, P. L. Nguyen, T. R. Rebbeck, and B. A. Mahal. 2019. "Conservative management of low-risk prostate cancer among young versus older men in the United States: Trends and outcomes from a novel national database." *Cancer* 125 (19): 3338–46. doi: 10.1002/cncr.32332.

McCaughan, E., and H. McKenna. 2007. "Never-ending making sense: Towards a substantive theory of the information-seeking behaviour of newly diagnosed cancer patients." *Journal of Clinical Nursing* 16 (11): 2096–104. doi: https://doi.org/10.1111/j.1365-2702.2006.01817.x.

Telang, J. M., B. R. Lane, M. L. Cher, D. C. Miller, and J. M. Dupree. 2017. "Prostate cancer family history and eligibility for active surveillance: A systematic review of the literature." *BJU International* 120 (4):464–467. doi: 10.1111/bju.13862.

Venderbos, L. D. F., S. Aluwini, M. J. Roobol, L. P. Bokhorst, E. Oomens, C. H. Bangma, and I. J. Korfage. 2017. "Long-term follow-up after active surveillance or curative treatment: quality-of-life outcomes of men with low-risk prostate cancer." *Quality of Life Research* 26 (6): 1635–45. doi: 10 .1007/s11136-017-1507-7.

Chapter Five

Radical Prostatectomy

"When It's Gone, There's No Need to Worry"

Surgery to remove the prostate gland seems like the most appropriate treatment for prostate cancer, but it comes with side effects that have a negative impact on quality of life. This chapter tells the story of a younger man with prostate cancer. He and his partner are in their early fifties with three children in high school. This chapter will tell the story of their experience of robotic surgery to remove the prostate and the challenges the couple encountered after his treatment.

Brent and Jamie met at college and were married the summer after he graduated. Brent is an architect and Jamie a nurse. They have three children, identical twin girls who are in their sophomore year of high school and a son in his freshman year. Jamie went back to work as an OR nurse once the kids finished middle school. They own a large home on a quiet street in the suburbs of a large city in the mid-West. The early years when the kids were young were busy, and Jamie is sometimes still resentful of what she sees as Brent's absence from their lives during that time when he was building his practice.

Just when things seemed to have settled down into a new rhythm with the kids in high school, Brent went for an insurance medical and found out a week later that his PSA was raised. This led to a cascade of doctor's visits, each one more invasive and more unsettling than the last. Finally, he heard the news he had been dreading: he had prostate cancer. But it was still in the early stage and the urologist recommended surgery the next week. Brent was not sure that was what he wanted; he had a big project to complete and didn't want to delay it. And he hadn't talked to Jamie about it; in fact, he hadn't told her about any of this.

Some men do not tell their spouse or partner what they are going through while being investigated for prostate cancer. This does not make much sense, but the most common reason is that the man doesn't want to worry them.

Late one Saturday night, just as they were falling asleep, Brent told Jamie that he was going to have surgery for prostate cancer and that he didn't want to talk about it or tell their children.

"Wait, what? What are you talking about? Cancer? Prostate cancer?" Jamie was dumbstruck. She was exhausted after a long shift that day and needed to get some sleep before work in the morning. "Hang on a minute. What do you mean?" Jamie sat up and switched on the bedside light. She was wide awake, and her heart was beating fast in her chest; she put her hand over her heart to try and slow it down.

"It's not a big deal," Brent mumbled, his back to her. "The doctor said I'd be in the hospital for a day or two."

"Brent! You can't do this to me! You can't just drop something like this and tell me you don't want to talk about it!"

"Jamie, please, I just can't, not now. Can we please go to sleep? We can talk about it in the morning."

There was no sleep for Jamie that night. She lay in bed, her mind a jumble of thoughts and feelings. How had this happened? Brent was just fifty-two years old; wasn't this a cancer that only old men got? It had been many years since she was in nursing school and, as an OR nurse, her work focused on caring for people who were, for most of their time with her, under anesthetic. There was a urologist who occasionally did prostate surgery in the OR suite where she worked; she would have to ask him how this could have happened to her husband.

Her alarm went off at 5:45 a.m., as it usually did on days when she had to go to work. She was exhausted and considered calling in sick but thought better of it. Her anger toward Brent had intensified as she lay awake and, to be honest, she was not sure what she would say to him. He was sleeping deeply as she dressed after her shower; she made no attempt to be quiet as she usually did, but there was no change in his position. She left the bedroom door open, silently wishing that one of the kids would wake him when they got up. But it was Sunday, and they might still be asleep when she got home mid-afternoon.

Jamie was distracted at work and one of the surgeons had to ask three times for an instrument. She was embarrassed about her lack of concentration and avoided the small talk in the break room between cases by sitting in the locker room, her back to the door, thoughts still swirling in her brain.

When she got home around 4 o'clock, Brent was not there. He had not left a note, and when she checked her phone, there was no message from him. Matt, their fourteen-year-old son, was the only one home. He didn't know where his father was either; Brent was not there when he got up that morning. It was not unusual for Brent to work on the weekend, but they usually talked about it the night before. He finally arrived home after 6 p.m. as Jamie was standing in front of the open refrigerator door wondering what she going to make for dinner.

Brent looked tired as he approached her, opening his arms to hug her. She moved out of his reach; she was so angry with him for not telling her about this.

"Jamie, love, I'm sorry. . . . I should have . . . I'm sorry. . . . Can we talk?"

She didn't know where to start. They had been together for twenty-five years, and things had not always been easy. She had struggled to get pregnant, and then the twins came. They were five weeks early and the first year had been so hard. Lilly, the oldest by three minutes, was stronger than Sophie and much more demanding. Sophie was small and the quiet one; she was not a great sleeper, and those early weeks and months had been a struggle. Then Matt came along, and looking after three little ones was harder than she had ever imagined. And all of this while Brent was starting his own firm. And now, this . . .

Matt came down to the kitchen and told them that he was not hungry and to not make dinner for him. Brent and Jamie were alone.

"Okay Brent, tell me everything and by that, I mean every little thing."

And Brent did. He recited what the urologist told him; he had something called intermediate-risk prostate cancer and he was told he should have surgery soon.

Surgery for prostate cancer, called a radical prostatectomy, is the choice made by many men and is usually
the one recommended by the urologist, a surgeon.

Jamie peppered him with questions. What stage was the cancer? Was
surgery the only treatment that had been recommended? Why had he
not discussed this with her before? He had no answer for the first two
questions; he did not recall much of the information from his appointment with the urologist, so he did not know the stage of the cancer.
He knew that the doctor, whose name was Dr. Bassett, wanted him to
have surgery, and he should know best, right? But he was busy with his
project at work and didn't want to take off time, and the doctor had said
that he would be off work anywhere from one to four weeks.

Jamie was furious with this statement and started to cry with frustration. How could he put his work ahead of his family? Had he even
considered the consequences of delaying treatment? And he had no
excuse for not telling her about this! She knew that he felt guilty about
not telling her at the time, but the truth was that he had hoped that this
was nothing to worry about and so did not want to worry her. Jamie was
perplexed by this; they were a couple and, before this, had shared everything. Life with three children was challenging on many levels, but they
worked things out eventually. Why was he trying to protect her now?

She wiped away the tears and took a deep breath. "So, are you going
to have the surgery This is important, Brent! You can't delay this. When
did the urologist say he was going to operate?"

Brent was not sure. He had another appointment with Dr. Bassett the
following week, but he was not sure what the appointment was for. He
had not asked the doctor about this; in fact, he had asked very few questions and had not done anything to find out more about the cancer or the
surgery. His work occupied all his focus these days, and the potential
of not being able to finish the big project he was working on scared
him. The project was worth a lot of money now and had the potential
for more work in the future. There were tight time lines on it, and Brent
could not hand it off to his only junior associate.

"Can I ask one of the urologists who operates at my hospital about
this? I think he knows the guy you saw, and I heard him say one time

that this Dr. Bassett is good . . . at least I think he was talking about the same person."

"Sure. Now, can we have dinner? I'm starving."

The next time Jamie worked at the hospital, she talked to one of the nurses she knew had worked in the OR at the other hospital where most cancer surgeries were done. The nurse knew Dr. Bassett and said he was a rising star and well respected by the other surgeons, despite being just two years out of training. The urologist who worked at their hospital was there that day, and she cornered him in the break room.

"I'm asking for a friend whose husband just got diagnosed."

What she heard concerned her; the doctor described the side effects of the surgery, but Brent had not said anything to her about this. She and Brent were both still young in her mind, and the thought of him having all the side effects the urologist told her about were very concerning. Why had Brent not said anything, and did he know about this?

It is very important that the partner of a man with prostate cancer attend all medical appointments with him.
They both need to hear the same information so that
there is no confusion or ignorance of the impacts of
treatment on the man that will also affect his partner.

When she got home from her shift at the hospital, she poured herself a large glass of wine and waited for Brent to come home. The twins were going to a study group to prepare for their upcoming exams and Matt was having dinner at a friend's house. Brent eyed her warily as he washed his hands at the kitchen sink. He was exhausted and didn't relish the idea of having a prolonged discussion with her about anything. He wanted to have some wine, take a shower, and eat dinner, in that order. But Jamie insisted on talking, and she had some questions that she wanted answered.

She told him that she had talked to her physician colleague, and he had said that robotic surgery was the way to go, but he had also described the side effects of the surgery. Did Brent know about these? Brent grunted in response to her questions. Dr. Bassett had told him about the side effects, and he was confident after talking to the doctor that none of that would happen to him. He was young and healthy, and the doctor sounded positive about the surgery.

"Why are you making such a fuss about this? Dr. Bassett is supposed to be the best out there and I trust him. He does this robotic surgery and I'll be out of the hospital the next day and back to my usual self within the week."

"I get that," responded Jamie, "But you are talking about the time immediately following the surgery. I'm concerned about the long-term effects . . . like incontinence and the sexual stuff."

"Oh that. Well, the doctor said that I should be fine. He's done a ton of these surgeries, and his patients all do great!"

Incontinence and sexual problems are the two side effects that impact quality of life after surgery (Mazariego et al. 2020). Incontinence has been reported by 15 percent of men after surgery and up to 87 percent of men reported erectile dysfunction at two years after surgery (Vernooij et al. 2020). Older men report poorer outcomes than their younger counterparts. (Preisser et al. 2020)

"Okay Brent, but the urologist I spoke to did not paint such a rosy picture."

"Well, perhaps he isn't all that great of a surgeon!"

There was no use in trying to persuade him to explore this any further, Jamie thought. "Can I at least come with you to meet this Dr. Bassett?"

Her urologist colleague had told her about the loss of bladder control after surgery, but she really wanted to know more about the sexual side effects of the treatment. She had done some reading on the internet, and what she found really bothered her. Some men never had erections again after the surgery, and she knew that this would be difficult for Brent to deal with. She wanted answers to these questions, and she would not rest until she received them.

"I guess you can. He said I'd be back to work within a week and that means I can meet the deadline for the project I'm working on. It's a big project, Jamie, you know how important it is for me."

Jamie went with Brent to his appointment later that week. Dr. Bassett looked younger than she imagined. He was dressed casually, wore small tortoiseshell rimmed glasses, and his hair was messy. But he was friendly, and he answered all her questions in detail. Brent seemed shocked at what might happen after surgery; he had not asked any questions at his first appointment with the surgeon and what he heard bothered him a lot. They had a great sexual relationship, he thought to himself, didn't they? Jamie asked about what could be done about the incontinence and the sexual problems and, at that point, he just blocked out their voices. This was way worse than he had imagined.

"I know this is a lot to hear and probably not as positive as you had perhaps thought." Dr. Bassett's face was serious as he spoke. "But we have to be realistic about things."

Jamie was listening intently, but all Brent heard was "blah blah blah." His head was spinning, and he really didn't want to hear about what this "reality" was that the urologist was talking about. The next thing he knew he was signing some forms and the doctor was shaking his hand and saying something about seeing him next week. He walked to the car in a daze and passed the car keys to Jamie; he was too distracted to drive.

Many men have unrealistic expectations of recovery after surgery and the reality of ongoing urinary and sexual side effects. It is important that, before surgery, men receive realistic and accurate information about immediate and longer-lasting side effects to temper their expectations.

Jamie tried talking to him in the car, but he said that he needed to get to work and could she please just concentrate on driving. When she dropped him off at his office, she watched him walk away, his posture telling her that he was unhappy. She tried to talk to him again before dinner, but once again he refused to tell her how he was feeling. She was worried about him; what Dr. Bassett had described was scary and she was not sure that Brent had heard much of it. Or maybe he had, and this was why he was acting this way. As the days went by, Brent withdrew more and more. He would not talk about his feelings, and Jamie grew more and more worried, and a little frustrated too. This was not happening only to him! She was going to be affected by what happened to him, too, but he seemed unaware of this, or perhaps he was ignoring her role in what could happen to them as a couple.

The day of the surgery came quickly. She knew from her experience as a nurse working in the operating suite that almost every person having surgery was anxious beforehand. She hoped that the nurses and anesthesiologist would be kind to Brent; she had asked around where she worked but no one she talked to knew anyone on the operating room staff at the hospital where Brent was to be admitted. She watched as Brent walked toward the changing rooms; he came out minutes later in a blue gown, his face grim and his eyes looking at the floor. He didn't even look back at her as the doors closed behind him. It was a strange sensation to be on the other side of the operating room doors, and sitting in the family room was unbearable. She walked up and down the hallway, counting her steps and trying to keep calm. She thought about going to the cafeteria to get coffee but was afraid to leave the area. So back and forth she went, up and down the hallway, waiting. She knew that eventually someone would come out to tell her that Brent's surgery was over, and she could see him in the recovery room in an hour or so; she had told so many families the exact same thing countless times. But it was different this time because *she* was the family.

Brent was groggy when she saw him in the recovery room. He looked pale, but this did not worry her, because she knew that many patients looked like this immediately after surgery. Dr. Bassett came to talk to them thirty minutes later. She could see that Brent was unable to take in most of what he said, but she took notes on a scrap of paper that the recovery room nurse gave to her. Brent's catheter could come out four days after the surgery; this surprised her a little as she thought the catheter should be in place for much longer. But perhaps things were different after the robotic surgery.

Brent came home the next day. He was weak, and the catheter was irritating, so he was grumpy most of the time. He slept a lot and was short with her when she tried to convince him that he should get out of bed and go for a walk. He still had the compression stockings that prevent blood clots on his legs, and she wouldn't take them off until he was more active. She tried her best to remain calm and not get angry when he refused to do what she told him to; after all, these were the instructions from the surgeon, and she was doing what she was told to, so why couldn't he do the same? On the third day that he was home, she removed the catheter as directed. It felt weird to do this for her husband; she was his wife and not his nurse! But she did it anyway and reminded him that this was almost as painful for her as it was for him. The worst part what that as soon as the catheter was out, he had a lot of urine leakage, and this was devastating for him. It wasn't just that day that he had leakage; the incontinence lasted for days and then weeks. He was not due to see the urologist for another three weeks, and he refused to call the doctor's office to make an earlier appointment.

Jamie had expected that he would have some problems after the surgery, but she was still upset when she saw how much this distressed him. She had taken two weeks off work to care for him and there were times when she regretted this; maybe she should have just left him at home because her presence did not seem to be helping. Any encouragement on her part for them to go for a walk resulted in Brent glaring at her and gesturing to his pelvic area.

"How am I am supposed to do anything with all of *this*? Diapers! At my age! This was *not* supposed to happen!" And back to their bedroom he went, slamming the door behind him.

> Bladder leakage (urinary incontinence) is distressing for men (Ilie et al. 2020) and may result in the man no longer participating in social activities, travel, and physical activity, and delaying his return to work. The man's expectations about return of bladder control will influence his response to ongoing difficulties, and embarrassment may prevent him from accessing help.

Things did not improve before they went to his first post-surgery appointment. Dr. Bassett entered the examination room with a big smile on his face; he looked confused when he saw Brent, who was sitting on the only chair, his body showing just how despondent he felt.

"Um . . . good morning . . . but it doesn't *look* like a good one. Tell me what's happening."

Brent looked up at the doctor and blinked, causing the tears in his eyes to roll down his face. He immediately brushed them away with his sleeve and gestured to Jamie to talk.

"Dr. Bassett," she began, aware that she needed to be careful with her choice of words. "Brent is having a lot of incontinence and, as you can see, he is not a happy man."

"I can see that, and frankly I'm surprised. The surgery went well, and his pathology looks great. But before we get to that, when you say 'incontinence' what do you mean?"

"What do you think she means?" Brent surprised himself at his outburst, "I mean, look at me! I'm fifty-two years old and I'm wearing a damn diaper!"

Dr. Bassett took a step back; he was shocked at Brent's outburst. "I see that you're upset, Brent, and I am sorry about that. I do need to know the details of your incontinence if I can help you. Can you tell me how many diapers you are wearing a day?"

Jamie interrupted, "He's changing about four times a day. He seems to do okay at night, but it's bad during the day."

"Hmmm," Dr. Bassett seemed surprised. "This is unusual after the robotic surgery."

I don't care how unusual it is, thought Brent, just figure out a way to fix this!

Incontinence has a negative impact on quality of life and may cause shame and powerlessness for some men. (Carrier 2018)

"I'm going to ask you to see a pelvic floor physiotherapist as soon as you can," Dr. Bassett continued. "My receptionist has her card. I'm told that she works wonders. And I'll see you again in another six weeks. Oh, here's a copy of the pathology from your surgery. We got it all. You should be very happy about that." And he was gone.

Brent and Jamie looked at each other. Jamie held the report the doctor had given her, and she passed it to Brent, who folded it and put it in his shirt pocket. He was not interested in reading anything right then. Physiotherapy? What help would that do? Jamie took the contact information from the receptionist on the way out. She called the clinic from the car on their way home, despite Brent telling her that it was useless and that he was going to have to find a way to live with the leakage.

"There's no harm in seeing the physiotherapist, Brent! What if it helps? Why are you being so negative?"

"Why do you think?" Brent muttered under his breath, but Jamie ignored him as she talked to the person who answered the phone at the physiotherapy office.

"That sounds great, thank you so much!" Jamie ended the call. "Brent, they have an opening tomorrow at noon! Isn't that fantastic?"

Brent grunted. He dropped Jamie off at their house and drove to his office. He was irritable and uncomfortable in the diaper, and he wanted this to be over. Why did he agree to the surgery? This is not what he expected, and he was mad at himself, at Dr. Bassett, and at the world.

His dark mood continued for the rest of the day, and he was grumpy when he got home. Jamie ignored him and reminded him just before they went to bed that he had an appointment the next day at the physiotherapist. Brent shrugged in response and lay on his side, his back toward her.

His mood was no better the next morning; Jamie tried to ignore him, but it was not easy. He complained about everything she did. The coffee was not hot enough, he couldn't find the book he had been reading, and he was behind at work and going to the physiotherapist was a waste of his time. Jamie focused on her breathing and didn't respond. They drove to his appointment in silence. She didn't really need to go with him, but she was not sure that he would go without her. She waited in the car while he was at the appointment and was surprised when he returned with a smile on his face.

"What happened in there?" she asked, "You're smiling!"

"The person who I saw was fantastic!" Brent seemed to have forgotten his reluctance to attend the appointment.

"Oh? What did she say?"

Brent told her what he had learned. For the first time since the catheter had been removed, he seemed hopeful. The physiotherapist was not just any ordinary physiotherapist but specialized in pelvic floor problems. Jamie sighed; that was what the urologist had said, but Brent was talking about this as if it had been his idea all along. But if this was going to help him, she would be supportive.

Incontinence after radical prostatectomy can take
some time to resolve, and men are often depressed
when dealing with this. Pelvic floor physiotherapists
can be very helpful in managing this.

Brent did the pelvic floor exercises exactly as the physiotherapist suggested. His mood was much better as he experienced less leakage and, within two or three weeks, he was no longer wearing a diaper. Life was almost back to normal, except for one thing: their sex life was nonexistent. Brent had noticed that he no longer woke up with an erection, and even thinking about sex did not produce his normal response. This was a big change for him, and one that he should have known might happen. Dr. Bassett had talked about this, but Brent didn't really listen. He was in shock and, anyway, he thought this was more likely to happen with older men. He was in his early fifties, after all.

He didn't talk to Jamie about this, and she didn't talk to him either. The silence put them both on edge and neither made any attempt to communicate what they were feeling and thinking. Their teenage children could feel the tension in the house, and they were not sure what was happening with their parents, so they stayed away as much as they could. It was not a happy home.

Masculine self-image is impacted by the loss of erectile function, and this can lead to distancing from the
partner and feeling diminished. Men may think that
the surgeon hid the realities of sexual problems after
surgery, and when they don't recover sexual function,
they feel betrayed.

Jamie was worried, so she plucked up all her courage and planned to ask Dr. Black, the urologist she had talked to before Brent had his surgery. He had mentioned that there were sexual side effects of the surgery, but Jamie had not wanted to ask for details; she had pretended that she was asking for a friend and it would be weird to ask for details. This time when she bumped into the urologist, she asked if they could find somewhere private to talk. They met on the stairwell behind the operating suite; this did not help Jamie feel comfortable at all, but she needed to talk.

The urologist confirmed that what she and Brent were going through was not uncommon. "Do want to hear the details?" he asked.

"Not really, but I should know."

What he told her was shocking; Jamie had no idea about any of the side effects he described, and she wondered if Brent had been told any of this.

Problems achieving and/or maintaining an erection after prostate surgery are common and most men will be warned about this by their urologist.

Jamie drove home after her shift, mentally rehearsing what she would say to her husband when he got home. She was nervous, as they had never needed to talk about sex before. Sex had always been good for them, even when the kids were little. Jamie had listened as her friends complained about their sex lives, but none of their problems were her problems. She used to wonder why these women were complaining to each other rather than talking to their husbands, but now *she* was hesitant to talk to Brent.

Brent came home a little earlier than usual and Jamie took this as an opportunity to tell him about her conversation with the urologist. She opened a beer for him and poured a glass of wine for herself while he was changing out of his work clothes.

"What's going on here?" Brent asked when he saw the drinks on the kitchen table.

"Can we talk, Brent?" Jamie's nervousness was evident in her voice.

"Sure, I mean, is something wrong?"

"Let's go outside where we won't be disturbed." Jamie opened the door to the back deck.

"Am I in trouble?" Brent was not sure what they needed to talk about.

"Brent . . ." Jamie took a big gulp of her wine, "I talked to Jim Black, the urologist that does surgery at my hospital . . . you remember that I talked to him before?"

"Yes, but what does he have to do with either of us?" Brent was on the defensive.

"Brent don't get mad, please. You know that things have not been the same between us since your surgery! You never touch me anymore and we haven't . . . you know . . . we haven't made love since before your surgery! I miss it, I miss you." Jamie tried to stop herself from crying. Her hands were clenched in her lap and she desperately wanted to touch Brent's arm, but she was scared that he would pull away from her.

Brent stared at her, his face reflecting a range of emotions that he couldn't put into words. Once she had started talking, Jamie could not stop.

"Jim told me what can happen to a man after the surgery and . . . did Dr. Bassett talk to you about this? Is that what's wrong? Please talk to me, Brent!"

Men often feel less masculine and regard themselves as a failure when they cannot perform sexually; this then impacts other aspects of couples' relationship. If these feelings are not shared, these couples may drift apart due to misunderstandings and false assumptions.

Brent opened up to his wife in a way that he had not done since he was diagnosed. He told her everything—how distressed he was when he was incontinent and how angry he was about his inability to get an erection.

Satisfaction with the man's sex life may take a long time to improve and medication alone may not be enough to help him adjust to his new reality (Albers et al. 2021) It is also vital that the man's partner is in-cluded in all discussions about sexual recovery (Loeb et al. 2020).

"Don't you think you should talk to Dr. Bassett about this?" Jamie asked. She didn't want Brent to waste any more time. Based on what she had been told that morning by her urologist colleague, the sooner Brent did something, the better.

"I guess." was his response.

Jamie sighed; why was he so reluctant to take care of himself? "Come on, Brent! You need to do this, for you but also for us! Don't you miss what we used to have?"

"Okay, okay, I'll do it. I'll call him tomorrow, I promise."

"You'll forget tomorrow or say you didn't have time!"

But Brent did call the urologist's office the next day. He and Jamie saw him later that week. Dr. Bassett was surprised when they told him that they had not received any information, much less a prescription, for medication that Brent could take. The urologist quickly printed a prescription for Brent and gave him some samples of the medication along with a pamphlet about how to take the medication. The appointment lasted about five minutes, and it was clear to the couple that the doctor was busy and didn't have much time for them.

"So much for that," Brent mumbled as they walked back to their car.

"Don't give up, Brent," Jamie tried to encourage him, "You have the pills and the instructions, and we can look for more information on the internet if we need to. And I guess I can ask Dr. Black for his advice. I feel like I should be paying him after everything he's done for us!"

Men with prostate cancer and their partners should have a discussion of sexual side effects before treatment as well as information about the emotional impact of these side effects (Mehta et al. 2019). Men often don't ask for help with sexual problems and psychosocial help may be more effective than medical interventions (Hyde et al. 2021).

Despite their initial conversation, there was distance between them. Brent had started to come to bed later than Jamie, and she was too exhausted most nights to argue with him. When she tried to hug or kiss him, she felt his body tense. This bothered her a lot and she wanted to tell him how she felt, but she was afraid that he would take this the wrong way. She didn't want to pressure him about sex, or the lack of it in their relationship, as she knew this would make things worse. He had the prescription from the urologist, but Jamie was not sure that he had filled it. Why was he not interested in trying to make things better?

> For men who normally have a high level of desire, the inability to get or keep an erection may cause distress (Bravi et al. 2020) and he may lose desire to think about or have sex as a result. Loss of desire can be interpreted by the partner as a lack of interest in them personally.

Nothing much changed over the next few months. Brent tried to hide his frustration with the lack of progress in his sexual recovery and Jamie tried to pretend that nothing was wrong. She wanted him to get help with this, but she was afraid to make any suggestions, because she knew he would react negatively. They didn't talk about what was happening, and the distance between them grew greater with each passing week. Eventually Jamie had had enough; they were going on vacation without the kids, and staying in a hotel had always resulted in more frequent sex. But with what had happened to him, she was pretty sure that this was not going to be possible.

"I don't understand why you're not doing anything about this situation," she burst out one evening just before she went upstairs to bed. "We're going on vacation and, well, what's the point if we can't . . . you know . . ."

"This again!" Brent responded as she feared, "Why can't you just let this go?"

"I can't let this go because it's interfering in our relationship, and if you can't see that, then you're more out of touch than I imagined!" Jamie tried to keep her voice down, but she was exasperated with him and the situation. "You need to get some help with this! Don't you miss what we had? Can you honestly tell me you're happy with our sex life? Or rather our *lack* of sex?"

Instead of arguing with her, Brent put his hands over his face, his shoulders shaking. Was he crying? Jamie put her hand on his back, and he turned around and buried his face in her neck. He was crying, really sobbing, and Jamie immediately felt guilty.

"Stop, love, stop crying! We'll get through this, it doesn't matter." She knew she was not telling the truth—it did matter—but she had never seen him so upset. "We'll get help for this, there must be help!" Jamie tried to console him, but she felt helpless and not just a little hopeless too. How had it come to this?

The next morning, Jamie searched online for information about erectile dysfunction after prostate surgery. She was baffled as to why she had not done this before and surprised that Brent had not done this either; or had he?

Jamie called Dr. Bassett's office the next morning from the hospital and, in a firm voice, told the receptionist that she was calling for Dr. Bassett. The receptionist transferred the call immediately.

"Dr. Bassett. You remember Brent, your fifty-two-year-old patient who is not doing well, even months after you removed his prostate? Well, this is his wife, and I need some answers."

Dr. Bassett tried to remember who this patient was, but he had so many patients. "Um, sure. How are you? How can I help you? I have a couple of minutes before I need to leave for surgery."

"Brent is depressed and hopeless! He has no erections, no sex drive, and it's affecting our relationship! There has been zero improvement! What are you going to do to help us?" Jamie's voice was angry despite her best attempts to keep calm.

"I'm sorry to hear this. Very unusual for this to happen with my patients. I'll send off a referral to one of my colleagues, a sexual medicine doctor. You should receive a call within a couple of days. What did you say your husband's last name was?"

Jamie told him, and the call ended. She sat with her head in her hands for a few minutes, her eyes closed and her heart beating fast. Why was it so difficult to get help?

She told Brent about the call after dinner. He seemed in a much better mood and was not annoyed when she described her call with his urologist.

"It's not a problem, Jamie. I called my family doctor and he reminded me about the little blue pill that Dr Bassett prescribed and I picked them up from the drugstore on my way home. Ta-da!" Brent pulled the small blue box out of his pocket with a smile on his face. "See, it's all good! I don't know why I waited so long to get these! You wanna go upstairs? I'll take one now and then we have to wait about an hour."

Erectile problems are extremely common after radical prostatectomy, occurring in 14 to 90 percent of
men (Emanu et al. 2016). Robotic surgery has not
improved the situation despite marketing campaigns
suggesting that it would (Fode et al. 2013).

That first night that he took the pill did not go well. Brent struggled to
maintain his erection and, even though Jamie tried to tell him that it
didn't matter, he was frustrated and angry. He didn't want to try again
that weekend and the next, and soon they were back to where they were
after the surgery: no touching or communication, just avoidance and
sadness. Jamie didn't know what to do to reach her husband; he was
distant and irritable and spent more time at work than with his family.
One of the twins, Sophie, asked Jamie what was wrong with him. She
was closer to her dad than the other kids and was sensitive to his moods.
Jamie reassured their daughter that he was "fine" and that this was not
related to the cancer. This conversation alerted her to how Brent's behavior was affecting the whole family, even though the other kids had
not said anything.

I have to do something about this, we can't go on like this, she
thought to herself. But what? She couldn't talk to the urologist she
knew at the hospital; this was too personal, and she was not sure that he
could help with relationship issues.

Family members, especially children, are often acutely
aware that something is not right when their parents
are struggling. Denying that something is wrong may
increase their fear that the cancer is worse than they
were told.

Jamie searched online for any resources she could find that might be
helpful to them. She found a couple of websites that talked about the
importance of getting support for partners in a similar situation. The
websites offered counseling for the couple individually and together,

but she was not sure that Brent would be willing to go for counseling. But she was willing to do anything to help what had become a stressful situation. She and Brent were barely talking, and he had started sleeping on the couch in the den. When the kids were around, they pretended that everything was normal, even though it clearly wasn't. Jamie had never felt more alone in the years of their relationship. She was going to try this counseling; maybe it would help, because nothing else she had tried had made any difference. Things were a mess, and she was finding it hard to see a bright future for them.

CONCLUSION

Sexual changes after surgical treatment for prostate cancer are distressing for the man and his partner and can result in changes to the relationship that further compound distress. The attention to erectile function does not address the loss and grief that both members of the couple experience. Pills and devices may not help the couple maintain the emotional intimacy that is vital to relationship satisfaction. Communication is a key part of adapting to the reality of the man's sexuality, which encompasses his identity and self-image.

Reflective Questions

After reading this chapter:

- What did you learn from this story about the changes in relationships after surgical treatment for prostate cancer?
- What are you willing to do to resolve sexual problems in your relationship?
- What advice would you give to someone else about relationships after treatment?

REFERENCES

Albers, L. F., C. N. Tillier, E. van Muilekom, E. van Werkhoven, H. W. El-zevier, B. W. G. van Rhijn, H. G. van der Poel, and K. Hendricksen. 2021. "Sexual satisfaction in men suffering from erectile dysfunction after robot-assisted radical prostatectomy for prostate cancer: An observational study." *Journal of Sexual Medicine* 18 (2): 339–46. doi: 10.1016/j.jsxm.2020.11.011.

Bravi, C. A., A. Tin, F. Montorsi, J. P. Mulhall, J. A. Eastham, and A. J. Vickers. 2020. "Erectile function and sexual satisfaction: The importance of asking about sexual desire." *Journal of Sexual Medicine* 17 (2): 349–52. doi: 10.1016/j.jsxm.2019.09.024.

Carrier, J., D. Edwards, J. Harden. 2018. "Men's perceptions of the impact of the physical consequences of a radical prostatectomy on their quality of life: A qualitative systematic review." *JBI Database of Systematic Reviews and Implementation Reports* 16 (4): 892–972. doi: 10.11124/JBISRIR-2017 -003566.

Emanu, J. C., I. K. Avildsen, and C. J. Nelson. 2016. "Erectile dysfunction after radical prostatectomy: prevalence, medical treatments, and psychosocial interventions." *Current Opinion in Supportive and Palliative Care* 10 (1): 102–7. doi: 10.1097/SPC.0000000000000195.

Fode, M., D. A. Ohl, D. Ralph, and J. Sønksen. 2013. "Penile rehabilitation after radical prostatectomy: What the evidence really says." *BJU International* 112 (7): 998–1008. doi: 10.1111/bju.12228.

Hyde, M. K., M. Opozda, K. Laurie, A. D. Vincent, J. L. Oliffe, C. J. Nelson, J. Dunn, E. Chung, M. Gillman, R. P. Manecksha, G. Wittert, and S. K. Chambers. 2021. "Men's sexual help-seeking and care needs after radical prostatectomy or other non-hormonal, active prostate cancer treatments." *Support Care Cancer* 29 (5): 2699–711. doi: 10.1007/s00520-020-05775-5.

Ilie, G., J. White, R. Mason, R. Rendon, G. Bailly, J. Lawen, D. Bowes, N. Patil, D. Wilke, C. MacDonald, R. Rutledge, and D. Bell. 2020. "Current mental distress among men with a history of radical prostatectomy and related adverse correlates." *American Journal of Men's Health* 14 (5): 1557988320957535. doi: 10.1177/1557988320957535.

Loeb, S., C. A. Salter, C. J. Nelson, J. P. Mulhall, and D. Wittmann. 2020. "A call to arms: Increasing our understanding of the impact of prostate cancer on the sexual health of partners." *Journal of Sexual Medicine* 17 (3): 361–63. doi: 10.1016/j.jsxm.2019.11.262.

Mazariego, C. G., S. Egger, M. T. King, I. Juraskova, H. Woo, M. Berry, B. K. Armstrong, and D. P. Smith. 2020. "Fifteen year quality of life outcomes in men with localised prostate cancer: Population based Australian prospective study." *BMJ* 371: m3503. doi: 10.1136/bmj.m3503.

Mehta, A., C. E. Pollack, T. W. Gillespie, A. Duby, C. Carter, S. Thelen-Perry, and D. Witmann. 2019. "What patients and partners want in interventions that support sexual recovery after prostate cancer treatment: An exploratory convergent mixed methods study." *Sexual Medicine* 7 (2): 184–91. doi: 10 .1016/j.esxm.2019.01.002.

Preisser, F., E. Mazzone, S. Nazzani, S. Knipper, Z. Tian, P. Mandel, R. Pompe, F. Saad, F. Montorsi, S. F. Shariat, H. Huland, M. Graefen, D. Tilki, and P. I. Karakiewicz. 2020. "Impact of age on perioperative outcomes at radical prostatectomy: A population-based study." *European Urology Focus* 6 (6): 1213–19. doi: 10.1016/j.euf.2018.12.006.

Vernooij, R. W. M., R. Cremers, H. Jansen, D. M. Somford, L. A. Kiemeney, G. van Andel, B. P. Wijsman, M. B. Busstra, R. J. A. van Moorselaar, E. M. Wijnen, F. J. Pos, M. Hulshof, P. Hamberg, F. van den Berkmortel, C. A. Hulsbergen-van de Kaa, G. van Leenders, J. J. Fütterer, I. M. van Oort, and K. K. H. Aben. 2020. "Urinary incontinence and erectile dysfunction in patients with localized or locally advanced prostate cancer: A nationwide observational study." *Urologic Oncology* 38 (9): 735.e17–25. doi: 10.1016/j. urolonc.2020.05.022.

Chapter Six

Radiation Therapy
"What Other Options Are There?"

There are a variety of other treatment modalities for prostate cancer including new ways of providing this noninvasive treatment: radiation therapy. Radiation therapy is often the choice for older men with prostate cancer who wish to avoid the side effects of surgery. These treatments, however, have side effects of their own, which may have an impact on quality of life. In this chapter you will meet an older couple wherein the man has decided on radiation therapy to treat his cancer and has his wife's support. Their son, on the other hand, is insistent that his father should consider other treatments, and it has a negative impact on their father-son relationship as well as relationships with other family members.

John and Ruby Evans met in high school and have been together ever since. In their mid-seventies, they are as much in love as they were back then. Like many long-term relationships, they have been through a lot together. John is seventy-six years old and a Vietnam War veteran; he keeps his Purple Heart medal in the back of his bedside drawer and takes it out on Veterans Day for a quick polish. The memories of his time in service are painful for him despite his pride in having served his country. He had a heart attack seven years ago and since then has exercised every day and watches what he eats. His wife, Ruby, is a year younger than him and has had her own health issues. Ten years ago, she was treated for breast cancer and, try as she might to forget that time in her life, she remains vigilant about her health, just in case the cancer comes back. They have two sons: Bruce, fifty years old, married with two young adult daughters; and Chris, their younger son, aged forty-eight, who is married with no children.

John sees his cardiologist every six months; he started this shortly after recovering from the heart attack, and even though Dr. Morgan thinks that an annual visit is good enough, both John and Ruby insist that these more frequent visits are necessary. At his last visit, Dr. Morgan looked more serious than usual.

"Uh, John, one of your blood tests suggests that you need to see one of my colleagues."

John looked over at Ruby, who was sitting to his left. What did this mean?

"I don't think this is necessarily a big deal, but your PSA was raised and well, I think you need to see a radiation doctor. Dr. West is a great guy, I trust him, and I sent a referral to him last week when I got the result. His office will contact you shortly for an appointment."

John did not say much on the drive home. Both of his sons have tried to persuade him to give up his driver's license, but he won't hear one more word about this. That would mean that Ruby would have to drive them everywhere, and that was not worth considering! On the drive home, Ruby wanted to talk—she always wanted to talk!—but he didn't respond to her questions. What was this PSA and why was it raised? He had never heard about this, and why did he need to see this radiation doctor?

When they got home, Ruby made them some tea and called their oldest son, Bruce. He worked in some sort of IT company that had something to do with health care or hospitals and Ruby hoped that he would be able to give them some information.

"Don't bother him while he's at work!" John reached over to take the phone from her hand.

"You stand back, John! This is important! If he can't talk, he'll tell us. Leave me be!" Ruby turned her back on her husband and waited for their son to answer the call. When he did, he sounded rushed.

"Honey? Bruce? We just got back from your father's doctor and something's wrong. He has to see some other doctor because there was something wrong with one of his tests. The doctor said something about a PAS . . . or something like that . . . ."

"PAS? Do you mean PSA?" Bruce sounded worried.

"That's it!" John spoke loudly so that Bruce could hear.

"Oh, okay. . . . It might be nothing, but it's important that Dad see whoever he's been referred to. Listen. Mom, I'm sorry but I need to go into a meeting. I'll call you this evening when I have more time to talk. Is that okay?"

"Of course, dear. That's not a problem."

John was relieved that he didn't have to talk about this, at least for a while. The truth was that one of his friends had told him earlier that year that he had a test, this PAS or PSA thing, and then he landed up getting prostate cancer. If this is what came after having the test, then he was not having any of it! This friend had told him that he had a whole lot of other tests and ended up with surgery and, after that, his life was just not the same. John wanted none of that.

Bruce called while they were having dinner that evening. John motioned to Ruby that she should not answer the phone, but of course she did. She talked to her son as John kept on eating his dinner; couldn't it wait till he was finished? He heard his wife saying "uh-huh" several times, and she was nodding her head through the whole conversation.

"Thank goodness for Bruce!" Ruby sat down and started to eat as she passed on the information from their son. Bruce had explained what this PSA test was and why John needed to see another doctor. John shook his head as she continued to eat and talk at the same time. He could barely make out what she was saying but he sat there, not looking at her, as she went on and on. After five minutes, he got up, took his empty plate to the kitchen sink, and turned on the TV to watch the evening news.

While he may not have listened to much of what his wife said, he was not one to disagree with any doctor, so he went to the appointment with the radiation doctor. He had a biopsy that was not exactly pleasant and a few days later was told that he had prostate cancer. The doctor did not seem particularly concerned about this and told John that he needed to have a course of radiation treatment.

"Easy for him, I guess! It's not him that has cancer!" John muttered to himself as he drove home. Now he had to tell Ruby and Bruce and Chris.

Ruby took the news better than he expected, perhaps because of her past cancer diagnosis. She went into "organizer" mode and started making phone calls to women she knew whose husbands had prostate cancer. John was not pleased with this; he wanted to keep this private and told her to cease and desist with the calls. Bruce and Chris also took the news well. Bruce had talked to someone he knew who worked in one of the hospitals that used the IT company he was associated with.

"Okay, Dad," Bruce stood in their kitchen as if he was making some sort of presentation. "The guy I talked to said that you need to get this treated as soon as possible. Don't wait, don't hesitate. He also said that one of the docs that works at his hospital is the best surgeon in the state, and he offered to get you in to see him."

Chris did not say much; he was always the quieter of the two. He sat at the kitchen table, his arms crossed, observing.

"Now hang on there, Bruce" John was not about to take orders from his son. "This doctor that I saw, Dr. West is his name, said that I need to have radiation."

"But *my* guy said you should have the surgery!"

John and Bruce started to argue, and Ruby intervened. "Stop it, you two! This is not helping. Let me tell you what I think. After all, I actually had cancer."

Chris continued to watch what was going on, but now he had a small smile on his face. This is how it always went—his father and brother arguing about something that neither of them knew much about, his mother interrupting, and round and round they would go until all three got tired.

It is not unusual for family members to differ on what the man should do to treat his cancer; how everyone reacts and acts usually falls back on old communication patterns. Adult children often assume that they have the right to decide what their father should do, this may be insulting.

John stopped arguing with his son and ignored his wife. His years in the military had instilled in him respect for authority, and Dr. West was the authority in this case. He hadn't told his family that he had another appointment with him the following week, where he would learn more about what the doctor had recommended. And he was going to make up his own mind about what to do, and if the doctor said radiation, then radiation it was going to be!

His next appointment with the radiation oncologist went well, as far as John was concerned. He had the last appointment of the day and went alone. Dr. West spent a lot of time talking and explaining about the treatment he recommended. Thirty-six treatments sounded like a lot to John until Dr. West explained that each treatment took thirty minutes from the time that he entered the facility until the time he got his car back from the valet. John liked the sound of that! Dr. West sounded confident that the treatment would be effective, but, most of all, he had explained things so well that John trusted him. He signed consent for the treatment and left with a number of appointments over the next few weeks.

Now he just had to talk to his family.

Radiation therapy is a well-established treatment for prostate cancer that is provided in different ways with the aim of controlling the cancer and limiting side effects (Kamran and Zietman 2021). For low- and favorable intermediate-risk prostate cancer, it is usually given as the sole treatment; for unfavorable intermediate and high-risk prostate cancer, androgen deprivation therapy is usually added. (Kamran and D'Amico 2020)

Ruby seemed satisfied with her husband's explanation for deciding to have radiation therapy. When she was diagnosed with breast cancer, she was offered lumpectomy and radiation rather than surgical removal of the affected breast, and she was happy with her treatment. And she was still happy all these years later without any signs that the cancer had come back. Chris, their second son, did not express an opinion about his father's decision; this was just the way he was—happy to stand on the sidelines on any discussion or decision. He had always been like this, and neither of his parents were surprised.

Bruce, on the other hand, wanted even more involvement than his father thought necessary. He had taken it upon himself to do some research into the treatment options available to his dad. This involved a lot of time looking online for alternative treatments, and he had even called a couple of surgeons and radiation oncologists to ask their opinion! He didn't tell his parents that none of them was willing to express an opinion beyond suggesting that his father, the patient, needed to have confidence in the treating physician. Bruce told his parents that he had done some research and he thought that his father had not considered any other options.

John was not happy with what Bruce had done. Yes, he knew it was with the best of intentions, but it felt to him like Bruce thought he was stupid and not capable of making his own decisions. Before they got into another one of their arguments, Ruby stepped in.

"Bruce, this is your father's body and it's his decision! You didn't interfere when I had cancer!"

"Well, that was *years* ago!" Bruce responded. "And I didn't have the contacts that I have now! I'm only trying to help. Forgive me for giving a damn!"

There are different meanings for the word "research." According to the dictionary, the word means an investigation, study, exploration, or enquiry. Academics do research when they conduct a study of something; health care providers do clinical research when they compare one medication or intervention with another to see which is best for their patients.

Ruby tried to lower the tension in the room by offering a slice of her apple pie. This was a family favorite, and she hoped that the pie would be a distraction. It helped in the moment, and they were silent as she cut them each a slice and placed a scoop of vanilla ice cream on each plate. But she knew that the silence wouldn't last long, and she mentally prepared herself to be the referee in any further discussion about John's treatment.

As soon as the pie had been consumed, Bruce started up again. "Dad, why are you going with the first thing offered to you? Did this doctor even talk about other treatments? Why not surgery? Have you even seen a urologist? Have you talked to anyone who has had surgery? I just don't understand why you would go with the first person, the first doctor, that you talked to!"

"Bruce! Stop firing questions at your father! He has not done anything wrong, and you haven't even given him a chance to respond!" Ruby was losing patience with her son.

"Okay, okay," Bruce took a deep breath, "I'm just trying to help, that's all. He's my dad! I want him to have the best care, and I have contacts."

John stood up from his chair. He looked defeated, his shoulders slumped, and his eyes focused on his empty plate on the table. "Bruce, I know that you think you are doing the best for me. But I am an adult, and your father, and I think I deserve a little respect from you about my decision. You were not with me when I met with Dr. West, and you don't know what he told me. I have made my decision and that is that. I am going with Dr. West and the radiation treatment. Enough of your questions! It's done!"

His voice had risen toward the end of his response to his family, and now he looked tired. He kissed his wife on the cheek as he turned to leave the kitchen. Chris started to get up to follow his father, but John waved at him to keep away. This was Chris's way; he said nothing when his older brother was arguing his point and then tried to make his father feel better with a hug. John did not want anyone to try make him feel better; he really needed a nap after all that.

It can be damaging to family relationships when one person tries to impose their will or opinion on the others. And it is not uncommon for an adult child to try and convince their parent that they know better.

After the boys left the house, Ruby sat at the kitchen table, absently picking at the remains of the apple pie with her fork. A lot of what Bruce had said made Ruby question if John had really considered other options. She knew that she had to be careful about what she said to John. She didn't want to inflame the situation any further, but Bruce had made some good points. Maybe surgery would be better for her husband. After all, once the cancer was out of his body then he wouldn't have to worry about it, right?

She waited until John woke from his nap and then asked him if he wanted to go for a walk. They had always been able to sort things out when walking, and it seemed to her that they had a lot to work out. Their house bordered on a large park that had walking paths that meandered along the side of a small creek. Walking made talking easier for them; they did not need to make eye contact and that sure helped when feelings were close to the surface and, right now, they both had a lot of feelings.

"Let's go, honey! It's warm out so you don't need a sweater and no one's going to judge what you're wearing!" Ruby was having a hard time persuading John to shake off his nap and get going.

"Why is everyone telling me what to do today?" John grumbled as he put on his walking shoes. He felt out of sorts and wanted to do anything other than going for a walk. But he sensed that Ruby wanted to talk, and he knew that if they didn't talk, she would only get more insistent and they would end up arguing about something small. But he was tired of talking! Or maybe he was tired of everyone else talking!

They walked in silence down the drive and onto the street. Within minutes they were at the entrance to the park, and it was clear that there were a lot of people enjoying what was probably the last warm day of the fall. There were families with young children and babies in strollers, and some couples, just like them, wandering over the grass to the walking paths. Ruby was glad that the paths were busy; there was less chance of John raising his voice if there were other people around.

Before she could start the conversation, John stopped and looked at her. "I do not want to talk about what happened with the boys today! I have had just about enough with everyone giving their opinion about my treatment. I do want to thank you for what you said about Bruce and his endless questions that feel more like accusations to me."

Ruby took his hand and started to walk along the path. She *did* want to talk about his decision to have radiation, as he hadn't considered other options as far as she knew. "John, honey, I do need to talk to you about something."

John started to walk a little faster, and Ruby lost her grip on his hand.

"John please! We need to talk about this. Remember when I was diagnosed? We talked about *everything*, and it helped me a lot! I was going to have surgery and you helped me to understand that the radiation and the lumpectomy was just as good! You came with me to all my appointments and that also helped. But you have been so closed off about what is going on with you! It makes me scared and I don't know how I can help you or even if you want me to help!" Ruby was out of breath now. They were still walking faster than she liked and her emotions were high.

John stopped on the path and turned to her, almost tripping her. "What is it that you want, Ruby? How do you think that you can help me?"

Ruby was taken aback by his tone; why was she the enemy in this? She just wanted to feel that she was part of his life! "I guess it would help if I knew that you had talked about with the doctor."

"Do you think I'm lying to you about this?" John was on the defensive and his words hurt her.

"No, of course not! I feel uninformed, you know, out of the loop. What did the doctor tell you about the treatment? Is it like what I had? I don't know anything about what is going to happen and I'm your wife! I think I should know this!"

Ruby was starting to cry, and she hated that; she often, or, rather, always cried when they were talking about something serious. John hated it when she cried, so she blinked a couple of times to get the tears out of her eyes, and then she wiped her cheeks with the back of her hand.

"Could I maybe come and meet this doctor of yours? If I could ask some questions . . ." Her voice was wobbly, but at least she wasn't crying anymore.

John sighed. He hated it when she was upset, and he did feel a little guilty that he had not included her in any of his appointments. Maybe it wouldn't hurt to have her meet Dr. West. They continued to walk, this time at a pace that was comfortable for Ruby, and by the time they left the park, they were holding hands again. The next morning, he called Dr. West's office and made another appointment for the following Monday, and this time Ruby would be with him.

Dr. West welcomed them both into his office. John had only seen the examination room and he was impressed by what he saw. There was a very large computer monitor on the doctor's desk and the walls were covered in certificates and framed copies of what looked like magazine articles about the doctor.

"You seem quite famous, Doc!" John was trying his best to control his nerves, because he was not sure how this appointment was going to go. He hoped that Ruby was not going to cry.

Dr. West smiled in response to the comment and motioned for the couple to sit down. "It's nice to meet you, Mrs. umm, Evans. Pardon me, I didn't forget your name it's just . . ."

"It's not a problem Dr. West. No one calls me Mrs. these days! Please call me Ruby."

"Thank you, Ruby. So how can I help you today? I'm very glad that you came with John to this appointment. I really like to have the partner involved, so please, go ahead with any questions or concerns that may have."

Ruby looked at John who, to his credit, looked embarrassed. "I have a lot of questions about John's cancer and the treatment he's going to have. I wrote them down if you give me just a moment to find the paper."

John was shocked; when did she write down these questions? And why didn't she tell him that she had done this. But then again, he hadn't exactly told her everything.

"So, our older son Bruce, he's in IT with some sort of hospital connections, and he wants to know why John has not been offered the operation."

"Ah, yes, the surgery question!" Dr. West smiled at her as if he had heard this question many times before. "Frankly, Mrs. . . . err, Ruby, your husband is too old to have surgery."

Too old? This was a shocker to John. He had just turned seventy-six and was fit for his age!

"Let me rephrase that! Because radiation therapy has as good outcomes as the surgery for prostate cancer, it is thought that a noninvasive treatment like radiation therapy is preferable because the surgery carries a lot of risks for older men."

This was something that both Ruby and John were not aware of, and they asked for more information. Dr. West explained things to them in simple terms, and they found themselves nodding as he talked.

"But what about side effects? And is the radiation really as effective in curing the cancer?" Ruby had both these questions on her list.

There is no evidence that either surgery or radiation therapy is the best treatment for prostate cancer for most men, and the recommendation for each man is individualized, based on the stage and grade of the cancer, as well as personal preference.

Dr. West explained the side effects of the radiation treatment that he had recommended for John. "Starting about a third of the way to half-way into the radiation treatment, you may find that you need to pass urine more often, what we call 'frequency,' and you may need to go as soon as you feel the urge. These are both what we describe as irritative symptoms or side effects. The other side effect that may cause problems is irritation of the bowel; you may experience loose stools or diarrhea, but to prevent this, we ask that you eat a low-fiber diet for the duration of the treatment."

Ruby was writing this down on the paper where she had written her questions. She was able to get most of what he was saying written down, but she found it challenging to listen and write at the same time. "I hope I'm not missing something or getting it wrong," she thought to herself. Almost as if he had heard her thought, Dr. West stopped and asked if she needed him to pause or if she needed clarification. This impressed her; no wonder that John trusted him!

John cleared his throat, glanced at Ruby, and then asked a question that he thought might get Ruby mad at him. "Um, Doc, what about, you know, what about . . ."

"What about the sexual side effects?" Dr. West interrupted John to his relief.

Ruby looked up from her writing. Why on earth was he asking about this? It had been a while since they . . . he was seventy-six, after all! Why would he want to know about *that*?

"Ah, another important question!" said Dr. West with a smile. Here's what you need to know . . ."

Much to her discomfort—this was their private business—Dr. West explained how the radiation treatment could impact John's sexual performance.

Radiation therapy does impact sexual function in various ways; the greatest impact on erections is usually seen at six months after treatment, and then a gradual recovery over the next two years may occur. (Donovan et al. 2016)

Ruby felt herself blushing as Dr. West described the side effects. She had never heard some of the words he used spoken out loud, and she was not sure that John had either. She was very uncomfortable, but she tried to write down everything he said. She was not sure why she was doing this, because she had no intention of talking to anyone about this, not even her husband of fifty-plus years!

Dr. West stopped talking and she asked if they had more time with him because she had another question.

"Sure, go ahead. I want to answer all of your questions if I can."

"My son wanted me to ask you about something called SBRT. I don't know what that stands for, but why is John not having that treatment? And what about the seed therapy?" Ruby felt nervous asking the doctor these questions; she hoped he didn't think she was being too demanding.

"Yes, SBRT and brachytherapy. So, SBRT stands for stereotactic body radiation therapy. It's another way of giving radiation to the prostate. We give a shorter course of radiation in higher doses. So instead of the thirty-six treatments that we have planned for your husband over seven weeks, SBRT is given every other day for about two weeks. We are planning to start doing SBRT here in a couple of months, but it takes time to get the necessary equipment and to train the staff. I would rather that your husband get treatment sooner than that and so that is why I recommended that he have the external beam radiation treatment. Does that make sense?"

Ruby nodded.

"Now about the brachytherapy, or seed treatment, as you called it. This is a good treatment for men who are eligible, and we take into account certain factors, including the size of the man's prostate. In your husband's case, his prostate is just too small for us to be able to put in the seeds."

Ruby nodded again. She was impressed by this doctor's willingness to explain things to them and she wished that Bruce was there. "But what about side effects? Is there a difference between these treatments?"

John's interest had grown as Dr. West answered Ruby's questions. He was not sure that the doctor had told him all of this when he saw him alone.

"The side effects are essentially the same for all three kinds of radiation treatment. But there's really no point in going over them again because, as I said, you are not eligible for brachytherapy and we are not ready for SBRT here yet. So, any more questions?"

The side effects of the different kinds of radiation therapy are similar. See chapter 1 for a detailed discussion of the side effects.

Ruby checked her list to see if she had gone through all her questions. Dr. West had answered them all, and more! And John looked like he couldn't wait to get out of his chair.

"I think we've taken enough of Dr. West's time. How about we leave him to his busy day and head home? I need a nap!"

They didn't talk much in the car; Ruby stared out the window, deep in thought, and John hummed along to the radio that was tuned to a classical music station. When they got home, John settled himself into the rocking chair on the deck, his face turned toward the warm fall sun. Within minutes he was snoring gently, and Ruby closed the door to the house so that he would not be disturbed by her voice when she called Bruce and Chris.

Neither of their sons answered their phones, so she left messages for them. In reality, it didn't matter what they did or didn't say; she was satisfied with what the radiation oncologist had told them, and she wanted John to get started on his treatment as soon as possible. They usually spent a month or so in Florida in the winter, so the sooner he started the treatments, the better, as winter was coming soon. When Chris called her back, he didn't say much, as was his way. Bruce was curt with her and she wondered if he had taken offense that his father had not listened to his suggestions.

Once John had given the go-ahead to start the treatment, things got busy. He had a couple of appointments scheduled one after the other; the first to have gold markers placed in the prostate to guide the radiation, and the second to talk to a radiation therapist who gave him a binder where he was supposed to make notes about how he was feeling on a daily basis. There was also information about what he could and shouldn't eat, and he gave those to Ruby. Two weeks later he started his treatment.

He drove himself to the treatment center; Ruby was annoyed as this was one thing she could do to help, but he did not trust her driving.

"There's valet parking! I just get out my car, go into the building, down the elevator, and I'm right there! Twenty or thirty minutes later, if they're on time, I go up the elevator, through the doors, and, with any luck, my car is waiting for me. That's what I call great service!"

John seemed to be enjoying this, and Ruby was happy for him.

After about three weeks, John started to notice the urinary side effects that he had been told about. He was not happy about this and complained a lot. His biggest problem was that he liked to settle down in front of the TV and not move for hours as he watched shows on the History Channel. Now he needed to get up every thirty minutes to go to the bathroom, and often it was a false alarm; when he got there, the sensation of a full bladder had disappeared. Ruby encouraged him to call Dr. West about this, but he didn't want to "bother" the doctor. He also didn't want to tell the radiation therapists, those "lovely girls" as he called them, because they were so nice to him and he didn't want to seem ungrateful. All that was left for Ruby to do was to not get upset when he complained, and to limit his fluids after lunch so that he could hopefully get some uninterrupted sleep at night. He was also a little more tired than usual, so his afternoon catnap most days looked more like a short sleep.

The weeks went by and not much else changed; he was still tired, and he was still complaining about the "pee" issue. He still refused to talk to anyone who could help him, and Ruby gave up on arguing with him about this. He had the occasional episode of diarrhea, usually after eating nuts even though he had been told to avoid them. Ruby had always said that stubbornness was his worst character trait, and his behavior during treatment confirmed this.

Urinary side effects are common during radiation treatment for prostate cancer because the prostate lies just below the bladder. While the treatment is targeted at the prostate gland, it is not unusual for some of the bladder to be exposed to radiation and this is what causes the feeling of urgency and frequency.

Bruce was not interested in his father's complaints. He was irritated that his father had not explored other options besides radiation therapy. The treatment he seemed most interested in was proton therapy, but John had refused to even talk about that. Bruce was convinced that this was the way to go, but he could not change his father's mind. John thought it was crazy to spend that much money on a treatment that was not covered by his insurance, and he didn't want to travel to another state to have the proton therapy. And Dr. West had not talked about it as an option, so it probably was not a good treatment. Now that his father was complaining, Bruce felt justified in his opinion that he had not been listened to and so now did not have to offer any sympathy to his father.

Proton beam therapy is another noninvasive treatment that uses proton beams to target the prostate. An increasing number of facilities are able to offer this; the treatment is regarded as experimental and usually not covered by insurance.

Someone had also told Bruce about something called HIFU and another person had told him about cryotherapy. He had found some information on the internet about both these treatments, but he could not find a doctor who provided either treatment close to where his father and mother lived. He struggled to understand why his father was prepared to accept the first treatment that was offered to him, but he realized that his father was stubborn and once he decided about something, he would not change his mind.

There are other kinds of treatment for prostate cancer beyond radiation therapy, however, they may not be considered mainstream treatments by oncologists. Treatments such as HIFU (high intensity focused ultrasound) and cryotherapy (freezing the prostate) are two therapies that are safe, but there are few long-term studies of their effectiveness beyond a few years. (Hübner et a. 2018)

After seven weeks, John's treatment was completed. He was a little sad when he had his final session and admitted to the radiation therapists, the "lovely girls," that he would miss their daily visits. He had bought each of them a small gift, and Ruby had baked a couple of her apple pies for them to have at their lunch break. He handed the valet attendant a $20 bill as he got into his car for the last time (or that he hoped was the last time) and drove home. Ruby was waiting for him when he arrived, a warm apple pie on the table with a tub of his favorite vanilla ice cream. It was done, and now all he had to face was repairing his relationship with Bruce. They both thought this was going to be the hard part.

CONCLUSIONS

Radiation therapy, in all its different forms, is an effective noninvasive treatment for prostate cancer in men who have localized disease. It is not suitable for all men, but in older men it avoids the complications of surgery. It also has a role to play in treating prostate cancer that has recurred, and this will be discussed in the next chapter of this book.

Reflective Questions

After reading this chapter:

- What are the risks and benefits of radiation therapy over more invasive treatments such as radical prostatectomy?

- How would you talk to a family member who thinks that their opinion is more important than the treatment choice of the man who has cancer?
- How do you look for information and what do you do to make sure that the information you find is credible and accurate?

REFERENCES

Donovan, J. L., F. C. Hamdy, J. A. Lane, M. Mason, C. Metcalfe, E. Walsh, J. M. Blazeby, T. J. Peters, P. Holding, S. Bonnington, T. Lennon, L. Bradshaw, D. Cooper, P. Herbert, J. Howson, A. Jones, N. Lyons, E. Salter, P. Thompson, S. Tidball, J. Blaikie, C. Gray, P. Bollina, J. Catto, A. Doble, A. Doherty, D. Gillatt, R. Kockelbergh, H. Kynaston, A. Paul, P. Powell, S. Prescott, D. J. Rosario, E. Rowe, M. Davis, E. L. Turner, R. M. Martin, and D. E. Neal. 2016. "Patient-reported outcomes after monitoring, surgery, or radiotherapy for prostate cancer." *New England Journal of Medicine* 375 (15): 1425–37. doi: 10.1056/NEJMoa1606221.

Hübner, N., S. F. Shariat, and M. Remzi. 2018. "Focal therapy of prostate cancer." *Current Opinion in Urology* 28 (6): 550–54. doi: 10.1097/mou.0000000000000547.

Kamran, S. C., and A. L. Zietman. 2021. "Radiation treatment in prostate cancer: Covering the waterfront." *BJU International* n/a (n/a). doi: https://doi.org/10.1111/bju.15550.

Kamran, S. C., and A. V. D'Amico. 2020. "Radiation therapy for prostate cancer." *Hematology/Oncology Clinics of North America* 34 (1): 45–69. doi: 10.1016/j.hoc.2019.08.017.

Chapter Seven

When Cancer Recurs

"I Thought It Was Gone for Good"

Despite the effectiveness of the established treatments for prostate cancer, recurrence can occur and requires additional treatment, sometimes with no hope of being cured. Couples need to learn to live with the uncertainty of disease progression and the risk that comes with that. The couple in this chapter are two men in a same-sex relationship for forty years; the man with prostate cancer has seen his PSA rise over the two years following brachytherapy. He and his partner are scared about what the future holds and what this will do to their relationship.

Roger and Matthew have been in a relationship for the past forty years. They met in New York City at the beginning of the 1908s, fell in love, and have weathered many crises in their life together. The HIV/AIDS epidemic nearly broke them as they saw many of their friends become ill and die. The sadness of the losses pushed them both to the edge of deep depression, but they leaned on each other and slowly the sadness decreased. They moved to Minnesota and were married in 2015, days after the legalization of same-sex marriage in the United States. Neither have had a relationship with their family of origin since coming out as teenagers, but they have created a family of choice that stretches from coast to coast. They are both retired now; Roger, age sixty-nine, was a high-school drama teacher, and Matthew, age sixty-seven, worked as the wardrobe master for a ballet company.

Four years ago, Roger was diagnosed with low-risk prostate cancer. He opted to have brachytherapy in part because of the more favorable impact on sexual functioning. He has been vigilant about monitoring his PSA since then. When his radiation oncologist suggested that it was safe to have his PSA measured annually, Roger insisted that he keep to the six-month schedule. Unfortunately, his last two PSA results have shown that his PSA was rising, and this was not a good sign.

> Follow-up care after treatment for prostate cancer relies on the PSA test. There is no strong evidence as to how often this should occur; monitoring is generally done every three to six months for the first two years and then annually after that.

Matthew always waited for Roger to share any information from his doctor appointments. After all this time, he was confident that, if there was something that he needed to know, Roger would tell him. Roger had not said anything but, for the last two weeks, he had been strangely quiet. The two men had very different personalities; Matthew was outgoing and liked to be the center of attention, whether they were in private or at a social gathering. He would talk to other customers at the grocery store and on more than one occasion had brought a homeless young person to their condo for a shower and hot meal. This horrified Roger, who was the quiet one; he avoided social invitations and was happy for Matthew to go alone and then tell him all about it when he came home.

"We're the yin and yang couple" was the way they described themselves.

As quiet as Roger was, his silence over the past two weeks worried Matthew enough to ask him what was wrong.

"It's nothing," he replied, "Just some stuff I'm working through in my head."

This was not good enough for Matthew. "Let me in, Rog. You know what they say: a problem shared is a problem halved!"

"Who says I'm having a problem?"

"Okay, okay! But I'm here if you want to talk." Matthew was not sure that Roger would share anything until he was ready, and he knew from past experience that he might have to wait a long time to learn what was bothering his husband.

Roger maintained his silence over the next week, and Matthew grew more frustrated. "There is a big gap between privacy and downright stubbornness!" he thought to himself. But nothing changed, and they avoided talking to each other beyond the most mundane requests to pass the pepper or to ask about what to watch on TV. One day when Roger was in the shower, his cell phone rang. Matthew knew better than to answer it, but he did glance at the screen as he walked past. It was the doctor's office, so Matthew picked up the phone and took it to Roger who was just getting out of the shower.

"Why do you have my phone?" Roger's voice was angry.

"I thought it might be important, so I brought it to you. Forgive me for trying to help!"

Roger glared at him and slammed the bathroom door closed. Matthew stood on the other side of the door for a minute and he overheard the first few words that Roger said to whoever had called. It was Dr. Gentry, the radiation oncologist who had treated Roger. Matthew was torn; on one hand, he wanted to listen so that he could find out what Roger and the doctor were talking about. On the other hand, he felt guilty for eavesdropping on a private conversation. But the thing that really bothered him was that Roger was keeping something from him, and he was scared that it was something bad.

Roger came out of their bedroom about ten minutes later. His face was shiny from the shower and his hair, salt and pepper now, lay flat on his head.

Matthew looked at him, waiting for an apology for his angry retort.

Roger sat down on a chair across from Matthew who could see that he was struggling to say something. "Matt, I'm . . . well . . . I'm sorry for what I said just now. I've been weird for a couple of weeks. I know that you know that and I'm sorry for that too. But, well . . . you know how I am . . ."

Matthew didn't say anything. He reached out to touch Roger's hand but then changed his mind halfway. His hand hung there for a couple of seconds, but Roger seemed to not notice.

"The thing is . . . um . . . my PSA has been going up for the past while, and at first it didn't seem to be a big deal but now it *is* a big deal and Dr. Gentry wants me to have more tests."

Matthew had been watching Roger's face, and what he saw frightened him. It was obvious that Roger was scared. His jaw was clenched, and he didn't blink, but just stared at his clenched hands in his lap. Matthew started to ask him why he hadn't talked about this before; it had been some time that he had been keeping this a secret. But, instead, Matthew stood up, took the three steps to where Roger sat, and pulled his partner into a hug so hard that Roger had to push him away so that he could breathe.

"Matt, whoa . . . Give me a little room here." But his words were kind.

"So what are you, I mean *we* going to do now?" Matthew wanted Roger to understand that he was not alone in this.

"I guess I, *we*, need some more information. Do you still have that friend who's a librarian at that nursing school? Maybe they can help to get more information?"

"Yeah, I think she's still doing that. I'll text her and see. What are you looking for? Is there something specific or just information in general? Wait, let me text her and see if she's able to help, and then you can ask her for what you need." Matthew was so happy that Roger was letting him help in some way that he was about to overdo things. He got his phone, sent a short text, and minutes later, there was a *ping* as a response came in.

Librarians can be a big help in finding helpful information. These professionals are able to help people find what they are looking for, often faster than if you tried yourself. Searching the internet can be like going down a tunnel that has many branches and any of these can be a waste of time in getting to where you need to be.

"Hey Rog! Jenny answered! She's still at the nursing school and she wants to know how she can help. Do you want to call her?"

Roger was not sure that he was ready to let a stranger into his private life, but Matthew looked so pleased with himself that he agreed to call the librarian. He had never met her in person, but she had gone to the same high school as Matthew. He made himself a cup of coffee and a toasted bagel, took a deep breath, and used Matthew's phone to make the call.

"Hello! How lovely to hear from you! It's been ages." Jenny's voice sounded friendly and just a little too loud.

"Uh . . . it's not Matthew. It's his partner, I mean husband calling. My name is Roger."

"Oh, Roger! Sorry . . . I saw that it was Matthew's number . . . so I assumed. . . . Anyway, nice to meet you, Roger. How can I help you?"

Roger hesitated. He was not sure how much he had to tell her, and he was embarrassed to be talking to this stranger about something so personal. "I just need to know what the topic area is and if you want me to find the information for you, or if you need help finding the information that you need."

"Oh, okay, that helps." Roger replied. "I'm not sure this is your field . . . but I need information about . . . um . . . about prostate cancer."

"Okay, that's a big topic!" Jenny responded. "Can you narrow it down a little? Exactly what do you need or, rather, want to know about prostate cancer?"

Roger was silent. This was more difficult than he expected. "I need . . . I mean, I want to know about what happens after treatment. What I mean is, what does it mean if the cancer comes back?"

Jenny had more questions for Roger, but she could sense that the man on the phone was struggling. "Okay, so do you want to know about why the cancer is back?"

Roger hesitated; he was not sure what he wanted to know. Roger could barely get the words out. "It's about the cancer coming back after radiation."

"It may take me a day or so to weed through this. There is a *ton* of articles in the medical journals about this. It's a topic that I am often asked about. The students in the third year of nursing study urology and they always ask me to help them, so I know a little bit about this, but I'm not a nurse. Please remember that."

"Okay, thanks for clarifying that," Jenny was matter-of-fact, and this helped calm Roger.

"I'll get back to you when I have something for you. Can I text this number or do you want me to contact you directly?"

Roger wasn't sure what to do about this. Would Matt be mad if he asked Jenny to use his own number? He shook his head; why was he being so stupid about this? Matt needed to know what was going on, so he told Jenny to use Matt's phone number to contact him.

Even though he had been insistent that his PSA was measured more frequently than Dr. Gentry had suggested, telling Matthew and now Jenny made his situation more real and more frightening. Matthew had gone into the kitchen while Roger was talking to Jenny. He was grateful for this but also a little guilty that he had excluded his husband from something that he had every right to know about. As he entered the kitchen, he saw that Matt was standing at the sink, looking at the wall in front of him. He put his arms around his husband's waist and rested his head on Matt's shoulder.

"Thank you for being here for me even though I am the biggest idiot and most selfish man on earth. I love you, and I don't tell you that often enough."

Matt didn't reply but he squeezed Roger's hands that were around his waist. He hoped things would be better from then on. No more secrecy, no more silence; that's what he needed way more than apologies.

Two days later there was a text from Jenny. She had information for Roger, but it was a lot and she wanted to know how she could get it to him. Matt asked if she wanted to stop by for some coffee or a drink and, at the same time, hand over whatever she had found.

"Coffee would be great, Matt, but it needs to be decaf if I come by on my way home in the afternoon!"

She came over later that same day, carrying a pile of paper about four inches thick. This was more than Roger had expected, and he was intimidated by just how much she had found. Was he supposed to read all of that?

Jenny saw the look on his face and smiled at him. "I've organized everything into separate categories to help you. See . . . here are some papers about why the cancer comes back. And here are some about what treatments are offered if that happens. And then there are some about side effects and more about how to deal with any side effects. I'm not sure if that is what you wanted."

Roger thanked her; this was more than he thought he needed, but she was so kind to do this for him, someone that she didn't really know.

Matt hugged her quickly and pointed to the coffee he had made while she was talking to Matt.

"Come sit down. Roger looks like he needs a stiff drink, and to tell you the truth, so do I!"

He made himself a martini, straight up, and a Negroni for Roger. Jenny cupped her hands around the mug of coffee, and they chatted for a while. She and Matt had not seen each other since their twenty-five-year reunion, and they tried to include Roger in the conversation, but his mind was on the pile of papers on the coffee table.

After Jenny left, he started to read. Some of the content was way above his head and he put those to the side. But there were some print-outs from cancer centers that had information that was easy to understand. He had a sandwich for dinner, the plate beside him on the couch, his focus on reading rather than on what he was eating. From what he understood, what came next was more complicated than he realized.

A rise in the PSA after treatment suggests that there the cancer is actively dividing in the body. Because this is found on a blood test, it is called a biochemical recurrence. Further testing may identify where the cancer is and additional treatment is recommended.

Roger read the papers late into the night. Matthew offered to sit with him, but Roger waved him away. It was fascinating but also scary to read the information. Roger hoped he understood what he was reading; some of the language was very technical, and there were a lot of acronyms that he found confusing. At midnight he finally stopped reading. His eyes were dry, and he was exhausted. He had made a list of questions for Dr. Gentry; he set an alert on his phone to call his office in the morning to make an appointment.

Matthew hoped that he could go with Roger to the appointment, but he didn't want to assume anything, so he waited for Roger to invite him. Roger didn't say anything, but Matthew overheard him on the phone with the receptionist; the appointment was at the end of the day on the following Friday. Matthew made sure that he was at home that day, but still Roger didn't mention the appointment. Matthew's feelings were hurt, but he tried not to show Roger that he was upset. Soon after 3:30 p.m., Roger went to change out of his shorts and T-shirt.

"Aren't you going to change, Matt?" he shouted from the bedroom, "You need to look a bit more pulled together if you're coming with me!"

"It would have helped if you'd told me that I could go with," muttered Matthew as he walked toward the bedroom. His heart felt like it was bursting he was so happy to be included, but he was also bothered that he had been upset that Roger had not said anything about him going to the appointment too. They were dressed within a few minutes, and they laughed when the saw that they were wearing almost identical chinos and light blue shirts.

Dr. Gentry was running late, so they sat in the waiting room alone; even the receptionist had left for the day. She had reassured them that the doctor had not forgotten them, but he was on call and there was an emergency that he had to deal with. When he eventually entered the waiting room his hair was standing up, and his white coat was ruffled.

"I am *so* sorry I'm late! Emergency that had to be dealt with . . . come on in . . . and just give me a moment to catch my breath! I ran all the way up the stairs, and I guess I'm not as fit as I thought I was!"

Matthew and Roger followed him into his office and watched as he took off his white coat and ran his hands over his head in an attempt to flatten the strands of hair that were standing up. He sighed as he lost that fight and sat down heavily in his chair.

"Okay, I'm here and ready to listen. What can I do to help you, Roger and . . ."

"Oh sorry, Dr. Gentry. This is Matthew. He's my husband, who I have pretty much kept out of all this. But I have seen the error of my ways and I know he needs to be here."

Matthew squeezed Roger's hand. It felt good to be part of this, even though the reason for the appointment was not a happy one.

Roger opened the folder he held in his other hand, cleared his throat, and began. "Dr. Gentry, I've done some reading and I have a list of questions. Is it okay if I start at the beginning?"

"Sure, go ahead," said the doctor as he leaned back in his chair.

It's a good idea to request an appointment specifically to ask the doctor questions. This is often a conversation that requires time, and the doctor may not have sufficient time during a regular appointment to respond to questions or to have a detailed discussion. It is also important to have a list of questions written down. In the moment, it is common to forget what questions you have and/or what information you need, and a list helps to focus the conversation.

Dr. Gentry listened as Roger asked his questions, and then answered them one by one. Roger sounded so knowledgeable, but of course this was not surprising because he had been a high school teacher before he retired.

The doctor explained why he had ordered more tests for Roger and also what he was thinking about as a plan. "Certainly, the rising PSA suggests that something is going on, but while I want to treat you quickly if this is indeed a recurrence, I also don't want to overtreat you if this is just a blip."

"But why do we, I mean, you not just go ahead and get it out?" Matthew was not sure where the words came from, but he had definitely spoken out loud.

Dr. Gentry smiled but Roger stared at him, a look of horror on his face. What did Matthew think he was doing?

"That's a great question and one I get asked quite often. Surgery, and by that I mean a prostatectomy, is very difficult surgery after radiation therapy, even in experienced hands. There are other options that have been shown to be effective in managing a recurrence, but first we need to find out what is happening. I have ordered a bone scan as well as a new test, called a PSMA PET-CT scan, that is useful for men like Roger."

"I still don't see the reason to wait! I'm sorry Dr. Gentry, but if you wait, won't the cancer just go wild?" Matthew was upset, and he ignored Roger who was shaking his head at him.

"I can see that you are frustrated, and you are a great advocate for your husband, but we really do have to do these tests. One thing that you should know, and that I told Roger when his PSA first went up, is that the rise in his PSA is slow and I am not particularly worried about this. But I do want to make sure . . ."

"You knew that the doctor was not concerned?" Now it was Matthew's turn to glare at his partner. "I have been out of my mind with worry! I thought the cancer was gone for good! Everyone said that brachytherapy was a great treatment!"

Roger looked a little embarrassed. He did not remember the exact words that Dr. Gentry had used when they talked on the phone. He was worried too and not sure why the doctor was not moving things along more quickly.

When the PSA rises after treatment, it is important
to be able to see if this is a local recurrence (in the
prostate that has been radiated or in the tissues close to
the gland) or a distant recurrence (in the bones). This
makes a big difference in what treatment is offered to
the man.

Both men looked at Dr. Gentry as if waiting for him to say something.

"Oh, yes, you had two PSA tests six months apart, and there was a
small rise. It went from 0.1 to 0.16. I am most concerned about the PSA
rising much faster. I have ordered the additional tests and, based on
that, we will have another appointment. I am being cautious here, but I
understand that you are worried." The doctor glanced at his watch and
Roger noticed this. They had been there for almost forty-five minutes,
and Roger was hungry. His questions had been answered and he just
had to wait for the tests and then again for the results. He stood up,
gestured to Matthew to do the same, thanked the doctor, and walked
toward the door.

In the car going home, they hardly talked. Matthew kept looking at
Roger who stared ahead, his focus on the road as he drove. Matthew
desperately wanted to talk about the appointment, but he knew that
when Roger went quiet like this, pushing him to talk was futile.

Roger had a bone scan one week later and the PSMA test the week
after that. Matthew wanted to go with him to these tests, to drive him
there and back, and to offer support by waiting with him. Roger refused
all his requests and grew quieter and quieter; ultimately, the couple was
once again barely talking.

About a week after the last test, Roger received a call from the radiation oncologist's office. Dr. Gentry wanted him to come to the clinic to
discuss the test results.

"Can't you tell me over the phone, Dr. Gentry?" Roger sounded
worried.

"I want to be able to show you the images so, no, we need to do this
in person tomorrow," was the doctor's response.

Roger sighed; this did not sound like things were okay. His heart was
beating fast, and he felt like he needed to throw up. He wasn't sure how

to tell Matthew about this, but he knew he had to. He was scared, and he needed support, and the last time he kept this from Matthew it was not good. This time he didn't wait; he went straight up to his husband, who was preparing dinner, and told him everything. He was on the verge of tears, something unusual for him, as he told Matthew about the call and the appointment for the next day.

Matthew hugged him; there was no need to say anything, they just needed to get through the night, and the next day they would hear what the test results showed and what would come after that. The wait was going to be difficult, perhaps even more difficult than waiting to hear about the biopsy results four years ago.

They were almost thirty minutes early for the appointment with Dr. Gentry. While they were sitting in the waiting room, a man came over to them and introduced himself as Miles, a physician assistant, who worked with Dr. Gentry. He told them that he would be with Dr. Gentry at Roger's appointment. Roger grabbed Matthew's hand as he explained this; it sounded like what was coming was going to be bad news.

Dr. Gentry did not waste any time with pleasantries after Roger and Matthew and the physician assistant entered his office. "The PSMA test showed a small lesion near the bowel, Roger. I don't think you need to panic, but I am going to suggest that we treat that. On the other hand, the bone scan is clear and that is good news. I know that this is not what you were hoping for, but this is treatable, and I would like to go ahead with that soon. You must have questions, so I am going to let you ask those."

Both Roger and Matthew were quiet for a few minutes. Miles, the physician assistant, started to talk but Dr. Gentry motioned for him to stop. The radiation oncologist had been in this situation before, and he understood that the two men, Roger in particular, needed a few minutes to gather their thoughts.

"Okay, let's get this going. What do I need to do?" Roger's voice suggested that he was less confident than his words.

"I think we need to do some targeted radiation to that lesion. It's really small, and I am concerned about how close it is to the bowel, but that is not something that you can do anything about. I am going to work closely with our radiation physicists to limit the potential damage to the bowel. Now Miles, here, is going to walk you through what comes next." And with that, he left the room.

Miles once again started to talk, but Matthew interrupted.

"Can we do this another day? I don't mean to be rude, but I think we need some time to let this sink in." He didn't look at Roger when he said this, but Roger did not say anything. Miles seemed a little surprised and perhaps also offended, but he didn't try to persuade them to stay any longer. He walked with them to the entrance, handing Roger his business card as they walked in silence.

Matthew put out his hand to take the car keys from Roger, who handed them over with no argument. This itself was unusual, because Roger always wanted to drive. At home, Matthew called their favorite Chinese restaurant to have dinner delivered and put a bottle of wine in the freezer to chill. The night required something stronger than their usual sparkling water.

After the food arrived, they ate in silence until Roger spoke. "Do you think I made a mistake by not having surgery in the first place?"

Matthew was not sure if he was supposed to respond, so he kept silent.

"I mean, maybe I should have listened to you and everyone else who said that surgery would take care of the cancer and then I wouldn't have to worry. But no, I knew better and had the brachytherapy! And all because I was worried that our sex life would suffer! Why did I do that? I think I made a terrible mistake!"

Matthew did not know what to say. Yes, he had thought that the surgery was better, but Roger had told him that the doctor had said that the risk of the cancer coming back was essentially the same for both surgery and radiation therapy, including brachytherapy, but had fewer sexual side effects. Now Roger, his beloved husband, seemed to be regretting his choice of treatment. How was he supposed to respond?

Regret about treatment, sometimes called decisional regret, is not uncommon. This is often related to the information provided to the man during treatment decision-making, as well as the source and amount of information provided.

They talked late into the night, their dinner growing cold and congealed in the take-out containers. The bottle of wine was left half empty on the table. Roger was completely honest about everything he was feeling. He was despondent about the side effects on his sex life that he was experiencing, and he was scared that any further treatment would make things worse. He was scared that Matthew was going to leave if they could not have sex again.

"I don't know about the side effects of more radiation, but one thing I am sure of is that I am not going to leave you. Not now, not ever. We have forty years of history together, and we've been through a lot. I love you and we will get through this too. And just FYI, I am not about to start training a new guy after all the energy I've had to put into training you!"

That made Roger laugh; not the belly laugh that always made Matthew so happy, but a noise that sounded more like a cough, but for Matthew it was enough. Neither man slept well that night but for different reasons. Roger's head was full of questions that had not been asked or answered about more radiation. Matthew could not stop thinking about Roger and his suffering that only now had been revealed.

The next morning, despite being exhausted, Roger began to take charge. He called Dr. Gentry's office and told the receptionist that he wanted to talk to him about the side effects of the radiation that he was going to have. The receptionist told him that Dr. Gentry was in clinic and not taking calls, but she would pass on the message to him. Twenty minutes later, Miles, the physician assistant, called back.

"Hello Roger. Dr Gentry is in clinic, but maybe I can answer any burning questions you have?"

"Well, I don't know, but here goes . . ."

Matthew pointed to his ear, suggesting to Roger that he wanted to hear and to put the phone on speaker mode.

"Hang on a second, Miles." Roger pushed a button on the screen and continued. "What can I expect from this additional radiation I'm going to have? I had some issues with burning when I peed after the brachytherapy, but it went away a couple of weeks later. What else do I have to put up with this time?" He sounded more aggressive than he meant to, but his despondency had morphed into irritation that he had to have more treatment.

Miles met his tone with a calm voice. "Everyone is different, Roger, but I don't expect that you will have any long-lasting side effects. The radiation is going to be targeted at the lesion, as Dr. Gentry said, and you may have some frequency, you know, the need to urinate more, for a few weeks. But the radiation is generally well tolerated."

Matthew moved closer to the phone. "What else can we do? It feels so helpless relying on just this one treatment. Are there vitamins or over-the-counter medications that can help?"

"Good question! Please be very careful about things that are advertised on the internet that promise way more than they can actually do. But some lifestyle changes can make a difference. And they don't cost money!" Miles talked for almost ten minutes about diet and exercise. Some of what he suggested were things that they were already doing, but the information about the importance of vigorous exercise was new to them. Matthew smiled as he listened; he felt proud that he had asked the question.

There are a number of lifestyle factors that appear to impact on progression of prostate cancer. They also have a positive impact on heart health that remains a significant threat to a man's health. Vigorous exercise and not smoking are two factors that are important after prostate cancer.

When Miles asked them if they had any questions, Roger answered that he had.

"I've been going to the gym three times a week for most of my adult life. Recently I've lost motivation but what you've said has made me think about going back. Is lifting weights a good plan?"

"Lifting weights should be part of your exercise routine, Roger, but the emphasis for heart health and your cancer should be vigorous exercise. Sweating, feeling your heart beating faster as well as breathing faster, are the hallmarks of vigorous exercise. Do you walk on the treadmill or outside at a fast pace?"

"No, not really . . ."

Roger looked at his husband, who was smiling like a cat who had eaten the cream. Roger had gained weight since he stopped going to the gym after the brachytherapy. Matthew had tried to encourage him to start up again, but he often said he was too tired. He avoided going to the gym even though Matthew continued to work out, usually three times a week. Matthew would never comment on his husband's weight gain, but he had noticed. Of course, he had. Roger had smoked the occasional cigarette in his twenties when it was still socially acceptable to smoke indoors, but had not touched a cigarette in more than forty years.

"I have another question . . ." Matthew glanced over at Roger. He wanted to ask about Viagra, but this was a sensitive topic for Roger, and he didn't want to upset him. Roger had started to have problems maintaining his erections. He was embarrassed about this and refused to discuss this with Matthew or his primary care provider. He bought some Viagra on the internet without telling Matthew, but his husband found the packet of pills in his sock drawer and made him talk about it. It felt good to clear the air, but the pills didn't help. After a few weeks, Roger stopped using them and their sex life ended, just like that.

Despite constant reassurance from Matthew that this was probably temporary or didn't matter, Roger had started going to bed later than his husband. He avoided sleeping close to Matthew and initially Matthew had joked that he was going to fall out of bed, but the joke was no longer even mildly funny. Matthew was hurt by this, and even more hurt that Roger didn't want to do anything about it. Roger had told Matthew that he was worried that using Viagra was connected to the recurrence of his cancer.

As you have read in previous chapters, sexual problems do not solve themselves and communication between partners is the first and. for many, the most important step in finding a solution. Not sharing feelings results in isolation on the part of the partner. Medications for erectile problems do not always work, or are not taken properly, and giving up without seeking professional help is not a good solution.

Both men felt better after speaking to Miles. Roger was reassured that he would manage any side effects, having undergone radiation in the form of brachytherapy before. Miles had also reassured Roger that the radiation would target the lesion that was seen on the scan and damage to other tissues would be minimized. Matthew was pleased that his thoughts about exercise were confirmed. He was going to get Roger out of the house and onto the treadmill at the gym, whatever it took. And he was going to make sure that Roger exercised vigorously too—he just had not figured out how to do that!

Roger started the radiation therapy a couple of weeks later. He was surprised to hear the radiation therapist talking about "salvage" radiation therapy. What did that mean? Was it something different from what Dr. Gentry had described? He asked Miles about this when he saw him after one of his treatment sessions. Miles was sitting with Matthew when Roger came out of the change room.

"What are you two cooking up?" He asked with a smile on his face. "Was Matt telling you how much weight I've lost since getting back to the gym? He seems really pleased with this despite saying that he didn't care what I looked like when I gained a pound or two!"

Matthew blushed and Miles laughed.

"He was telling me that he loves the fact that you go with him to the gym. And I can certainly see that you have lost weight! You look great!"

"Can I ask you a question, Miles?" Roger was bothered by the word "salvage"; it sounded like the situation was hopeless.

"Sure, what's up?"

"What does 'salvage' radiation therapy mean? The radiation therapist said that is what I'm having, and no one has mentioned that word before."

"Ah, the language of medicine. Salvage therapy is the term we use for treatment after a recurrence occurs. It's not a great word because it does sound ominous. There are other terms we use for radiation treatment too. For example, the term 'adjuvant' radiation means that the radiation is given after surgery for prostate cancer and is usually used for men with high-risk prostate cancer. There is also the term 'neoadjuvant radiation' where radiation is used before another kind of treatment."

Roger nodded his head as the physician assistant spoke. There was so much more to learn about this disease, and even though he had thought that it was behind him after his initial treatment, he knew that there was still more to learn. Taking care of his health was an important part of that, and even though he didn't want to admit it, he felt much better since he had started exercising again. And being more open with Matthew and sharing his feelings had also helped bring them closer. He wished that he didn't have to learn these lessons the hard way, but learning them was worthwhile.

CONCLUSION

Even though surgery and radiation are effective treatments for prostate cancer, there is a risk that the cancer will come back months or years later. Fortunately, more recurrences of the cancer are detected early because measuring the PSA after treatment is very useful for the detection of what is called a "biochemical recurrence." This means that the recurrence is found based on a rising PSA rather than on symptoms suggesting that the cancer has spread. Additional radiation therapy, or other treatments, can be effective in managing the recurrence.

Reflective Questions

After reading this chapter:

- How can a partner be supportive when the man with cancer finds it hard to talk about what he is going through?
- What strategies can be used to encourage the man to include exercise and a healthy diet in his daily life when he says he is too tired to exercise or doesn't want to make changes to his diet?
- How can a partner find answers to their questions about treatment without disclosing information about the man with prostate cancer?

Chapter Eight

Androgen Deprivation Therapy

"He's Not a Man Anymore"

Androgen deprivation therapy, a treatment that stops the man's body from producing testosterone, thus starving the prostate cancer cells of the fuel needed to survive, is prescribed for men with advanced or recurrent disease. This treatment has significant side effects that impact quality of life. In this chapter, readers will meet a couple who is dealing with the side effects of this treatment and the ensuing challenges to their relationship.

Ross and Margaret Adams have not had the easiest marriage. They are both stubborn and quick to anger but this does not mean they don't love each other; they do, deeply. And while their arguments were brief, they happened frequently and tended to involve sulking for a while afterward. But eventually, the couple would go back to their usual selves. They are both sixty-six years old and have been married for forty years, which is a long time for constant arguing! They have a son, Nolan, and a daughter, Ruth, neither of whom have ever married. This is the source of their greatest sadness. They would love to have grandchildren but given that Nolan and Ruth are both in their forties and unattached, this is not likely to happen.

Ross was diagnosed with high-risk prostate cancer—the news coming on his birthday. He had avoided medical care for most of his life, much to Margaret's disapproval, but one day he fainted at work and was taken to the closest emergency department by ambulance. Fortunately, it was not anything serious; he was dehydrated and his blood pressure was too high. Margaret insisted that he see her nurse practitioner at the drugstore close to their home. The nurse practitioner was very thorough and ordered a long list of blood tests for him. His PSA was high ("through the roof" Margaret said, although she had no frame of reference for this) and he saw a urologist within the month, had a biopsy, and received a diagnosis of prostate cancer. It was recommended that he have surgery to remove his prostate, but he flat-out refused. The thought of someone cutting into his body made him feel sick to his stomach. So he was referred to a radiation oncologist, who offered him radiation therapy. He saw the radiation oncologist, Dr. Wong, that same week, and the doctor did not waste his words.

"Ross, your cancer is not good. Your prostate is full of high-grade disease and, while I think we can manage it, cure may not be possible. I'm recommending an eight-week course of external beam radiation, and you are going to need at least two years of hormone therapy. You need some scans before we get going. If the cancer has already spread outside the prostate, then the whole plan changes. You okay with this?"

Ross was not sure what to say. He knew that he didn't want surgery, but he was not sure what the scans were and how they would make a difference. And what was hormone therapy?

Androgen deprivation therapy has been used for many years to treat men with advanced prostate cancer. It is commonly referred to as "hormone therapy" but this is an inaccurate term. Prostate cancer needs androgens or male hormones, namely testosterone and dihydrotestosterone, in order to grow, so the correct term for this therapy is androgen deprivation.

"Um, what scans, Doc? And what do you mean by the plans changing?" Ross's voice reflected his fear. His cancer was suddenly very real, and he wished that he had done some reading about it before this appointment.

"I want you to have a bone scan and a CT scan. Oh, and a repeat PSA. That'll give us a good idea of what the situation is and hopefully we can get started on the radiation soon. In the meantime, I am going to write you a prescription for a pill that I want you to take for a month before we start with the hormone therapy. Let me go and do that right now. You can think of any questions while I'm doing that."

Ross sat staring at a poster on the wall with a large diagram of the prostate gland. He hardly registered what he was looking at, his mind was a million miles away. After about ten minutes, Dr. Wong came back into the room.

"Okay, so I've ordered the tests and you will get a call from my receptionist with the dates and times for these scans. You can go down to the lab in this building to have the blood test right now, but it'll take a day or two before you get the other tests. Oh, here's the prescription for the pills I mentioned. Any questions?"

Ross shook his head. This was all too much, but what choice did he have? He liked Dr. Wong, the radiation oncologist. He was a little brusque, but Ross appreciated his honesty. His reception staff was very friendly, almost as if they knew they had to make up for his lack of bedside manner. He went downstairs to the lab, as instructed, and had blood drawn. He hardly felt the needle going into his vein; his thoughts were focused on what would happen if the cancer had spread, and he was very scared.

When he got home, Margaret asked him about the appointment. He told her that he needed more tests and then Dr. Wong would start the radiation. He didn't mention anything about the prescription in his pocket because he had forgotten all about it! Later that night as he hung up his pants, he heard the crinkle of paper and remembered that he needed to get the medication. He shook his head; he was usually not this forgetful.

Androgen deprivation therapy starts with two weeks or a month of pills, followed by injections every three, six, or twelve months.

Ross went to the drugstore early the next morning to get the prescription filled. He didn't tell his wife why or where he was going, and she didn't ask. She assumed he was sulking about something she may or may not have done and she knew that eventually he would tell her what was bothering him. But he didn't say a word and just went into the den and disappeared into a detective novel he was reading. Margaret peeked in on him every half hour or so, but he didn't even look up. This was so typical of him, she thought, leaving her to wonder and worry.

She hoped that he would talk to her during dinner, but he turned up the volume on the evening news and ignored her. After thirty minutes of hearing him chew, too loudly for her liking, and the droning of the newscaster, she had had enough.

"Are you ever going to talk to me?" her voice was loud. "What have I done to annoy you this time? Honestly, Ross, forty years is a long time for this nonsense! If I have done something to you, or maybe not done for you, just tell me and we can move on! I can't stand being ignored like this!"

"You haven't done anything! Can a man not eat in peace?"

Margaret did not respond. She didn't want to argue with him while he was dealing with the cancer, but she felt left out and was not sure when his treatment would start, or any of the details other than him needing more tests of some sort. She got up from the table, taking her half-full plate with her; she had no appetite when they were at odds.

Over the next few days, they barely spoke. Ross had the bone and CT scan that week, without mentioning where he was going as he left the house. This upset Margaret; she wanted to support him but how was she supposed to do that if he didn't tell her anything? She was not sure if he had told Nolan and Ruth about his diagnosis, so she couldn't even ask them for support as she struggled with his silence.

> While some couples draw closer together after a cancer diagnosis, other couples experience an exacerbation of their usual functioning, which leads to more silence, more arguments, and more distress.

Ross had another appointment with Dr. Wong the following week. He had started taking some pills that the doctor had prescribed, and he noticed that he had some swelling under his nipples. He thought this was weird, but he did not recall Dr. Wong mentioning this. What did this mean? He couldn't find the papers that came with the pills; he'd thrown them away when he got back from the drugstore and he now regretted not reading them. He didn't like looking up things on the internet and usually asked Margaret to do this, but he was reluctant to ask her this time. That would lead to a whole lot of questions about why he was taking the medication, and why hadn't he told her about this, and why was he so secretive. It would lead to a fight, and he was too tired to fight these days. He made a mental note to talk to Dr. Wong at his next appointment that was scheduled for the following Tuesday afternoon.

This time he asked Margaret to go with him to the appointment. Things had begun to thaw between them, just as they had for the decades of their marriage. It started slowly with Margaret baking his favorite carrot cake for seemingly no reason at all. They shared a slice after dinner one evening, and that led to a walk together along the river the next afternoon, and by the time they got home, they were holding hands. Margaret got tears in her eyes when Ross asked her to go with him to see Dr. Wong. She turned away so that he wouldn't see how much this meant to her.

Margaret was nervous the day of the appointment; she was not sure why, but it seemed that this was an important appointment and Ross looked a little apprehensive too. They didn't talk much on the drive there and were silent in the waiting room, but Margaret reached for her husband's hand and this calmed them both. They didn't have a long wait, less than five minutes, when the receptionist led them into Dr. Wong's office. They were not alone for long, as Dr. Wong entered the room just a minute later.

"Good afternoon, Ross! Is it okay if I call you by your first name?" Dr. Wong talked as he settled into his chair and started typing on the keyboard of his computer. "And who do you have with you today?" he asked as he looked up at Margaret.

"Oh, this is my wife, Margaret, Dr. Wong," Ross looked a little embarrassed as he introduced his spouse. He was a little afraid that the doctor was going to ask why he had not brought Margaret with him before, but the doctor didn't say anything and just smiled at Margaret.

"I have the results of your scans here, Ross. Everything looks good, so we can go ahead with the radiation. I'd like to start next week, so this is going to be a busy rest of the week for you. You need to have something we call a 'CT simulation,' and you also need to meet with one of the radiation therapists. All of this will happen at the cancer clinic next door to where you had the scans. Any questions?"

Margaret had a lot of questions, but she waited to see if Ross was going to say anything. She looked at him, and he had a strange expression on his face. He looked confused and this was unusual for him—he was so opinionated most of the time.

"Ross, did you hear what the doctor said?" Her voice was soft and not confrontational.

Ross shook his head; he seemed dazed.

"Do you have any questions, err . . . Margaret?" Dr. Wong looked at Ross as he said this.

He was surprised that his patient was so quiet. This was rather unusual because most men had a lot of questions, especially when he had just shared the results of scans.

"I do have questions, Dr. Wong, I have a lot of questions! I'm sorry to have to say this in front of your doctor, Ross, but I know almost nothing about these scans or pretty much anything else!" To her embarrassment, she was on the verge of tears at her outburst.

"Not to worry, Margaret, I'll explain everything as long as that's okay with your husband."

Ross did not say anything and shrugged his shoulders. Margaret was worried about his behavior, but she did not want to stop the doctor from telling her what was happening. She would deal with Ross later; now she needed to hear what Dr. Wong had to say.

She listened intently as the doctor explained things to her. He started at the beginning, with the biopsy results, then went into the radiation treatment that was planned as well as her husband's scans that, thankfully, showed that the cancer had not spread outside the prostate. He explained the androgen deprivation therapy that Ross had started with the pills for a month ("what pills?" Margaret wondered), and then the details of the radiation therapy over eight weeks and the three-monthly injections to lower his testosterone levels.

Margaret felt like her head was going to explode. This was a lot of information, almost all of it that was new to her. She was also annoyed—no, angry—with Ross for keeping this from her, and making her look stupid in front of his doctor.

Oncology providers are aware of the importance of outside support and should address this with the patient, should he come to appointments without a family member or friend. Contact information for the treating physician and all members of the treatment team should also be provided to someone other than the patient.

Margaret thanked the doctor for his time. She was appreciative that he had shared so much information with her, but she now needed to think about what he had told her. Her mind was reeling with what she had heard, and she needed to think about how she was going to get through to Ross that not telling her what was going on was not in his best interest. She was furious with him, but she also knew that being angry was not productive. They didn't talk on the way home, and this gave her some time to think about what she was going to say to him.

When they got home, she busied herself getting dinner ready. It was only 4 p.m., but she needed to do something or else she was going to blow up at her husband. She was not really focused on what she was doing, but opening and closing the cupboard doors and banging pots felt good. She hardly noticed that Ross was standing in the doorway, looking at her.

"What? What is it?" She glared at him, her hands on her hips.

To her surprise, Ross asked her if they could go for a walk. She felt all the air go out of her lungs, and in the same moment, most of her anger left her.

"Okay, where do you want to go?"

"Nowhere in particular," Ross replied, his voice so soft she could barely hear him. "I think we need to talk."

Margaret was about to respond, but she bit her lip and kept quiet. She turned off the oven, washed her hands, went to the foyer and put on her walking shoes. She waited for him at the front door while he tied his shoes. She noticed that he winced as he bent over and she immediately felt concerned. Was he in pain and did this mean something about the cancer?

"Ross, are you okay? You look like you're in pain."

"It's okay . . . well, not really . . . can we just talk about this as we walk?"

Margaret nodded, but she was worried. Two minutes later they were walking down the street, their footsteps crunching on the road.

Margaret waited for Ross to say something. He cleared his throat, but no words came out of his mouth. She found herself getting irritated but took a couple of deep breaths; she would just have to wait.

When they got the end of the street, Ross stopped walking. She was a few steps ahead of him when she realized that he was not at her side. She turned quickly and saw him standing still, his arms hanging by his side.

"What's wrong?" her voice was shrill, "Ross, are you okay? What is it?" She reached his side in what felt like a nanosecond. "Ross! Tell me! What are you feeling? Do I need to call 911?"

Ross shook his head. "I do want to talk about something," he was still talking softly, so Margaret had to stand close to him, close enough that he took her hand in his. "I know I've not told you much about what I'm going through."

Margaret almost laughed at this understatement, but she just looked at him, her eyebrows raised.

"Okay, okay, I pretty much haven't told you anything," Ross continued. "I guess I just needed time to wrap my head around all of this. You know those pills that Dr. Wong talked about?"

Margaret nodded her head.

"Well, I've been taking them and . . . this is so embarrassing . . . I've gone and developed . . . um, how do I say this? I've gotten boobs, and they hurt!"

He looked so uncomfortable saying the word "boobs" that Margaret smiled, but then felt bad about that. "Oh, Ross, I'm so sorry that you're in pain, but you don't have to be embarrassed! I noticed that you winced when you were tying your shoes, and now I know the reason." It felt so strange talking to her husband about this, but at least now things were out in the open and maybe he would talk about what else was bothering him.

Breast tenderness and swelling is one of the more common side effects of bicalutamide, the anti-androgen medication that is usually prescribed for men starting androgen deprivation therapy.

"Is that all?" she asked.

"Not really, but what else am I going to have to go through? I don't remember Dr. Wong talking about this breast thing, and I'm scared about what else could go wrong."

Ross was obviously distressed, and this made Margaret feel like she had to act like she was the strong one. "Now hang on a minute, here! This presumably is a side effect of the pills. I don't think this means that anything is going wrong. I didn't hear the doctor say anything about this when I was with you at the appointment, but maybe he thought that you had told me. Anyway, we can look this up on Google when we get home. I am also going to check what the side effects of the radiation are in case you . . . I mean we, didn't hear that either. What I do know is that we have to tell Nolan and Ruth about this."

"Do we have to? I'd rather we kept this just between us." Ross had the decency to look sheepish as he said this. But Margaret was having none of this.

"Your children are not babies! They are in their forties and even if you don't, I need their support as we go through the next months of your treatment! How do you think they'll feel when they find out that you have not told them something as important as this?" Margaret felt exasperated and it was hard to feel sympathetic when he was being this stubborn.

"I know, I know," Ross was almost pleading, "But could you please tell them? I don't think I have the strength."

Margaret shook her head; there was no use arguing with him when he got like this, and if she had to tell Nolan and Ruth because he refused to, that was better than not telling them at all. But she was going to make sure that he was there when she told them!

They turned around and walked back home, having covered less than half a block. Margaret went straight to the phone to call their two children while Ross turned on the TV and was snoring within minutes. Ross had been to two appointments that week and had mentioned that he was more tired than usual, so Margaret left him to nap on the couch. She covered him with the blanket they kept for afternoon naps and tried to make as little noise as possible as she prepared their dinner. He was due to start the radiation and she was determined that she was going to be as supportive as she could be, even though he didn't make things easy for her.

Margaret tried to sound normal when she invited first Ruth and then Nolan for Sunday lunch the next weekend. She was not feeling anywhere near normal, but her voice sounded fine in her ears. Both Ruth and Nolan asked if it was a special occasion and she lied and said that she and Ross missed them and wanted to spend some time with them. She told them she was making roast chicken and lemon potatoes, a favorite of theirs, and this was enough to stop the questions and the invitation was accepted.

They arrived bearing gifts. Nolan had purchased his father's favorite black licorice from a specialty store at the local market, and Ruth had a bunch of sunflowers that brightened the kitchen with their large brown centers and brilliant yellow petals. Margaret loved fresh flowers and Ruth knew how pleased she would be with these blooms. They sat down to eat within minutes, and there was not much conversation at first, beyond thanks from Nolan and Ruth for the delicious meal. Margaret worried about her adult children even though they were quite capable of taking care of themselves. They both worked hard in their respective jobs, and she was sure that they didn't eat properly; cooking for them was part pleasure and part assurance about their nutrition. Soon their plates were empty and smeared with the last of the juices from the potatoes.

Margaret looked at her husband, her expression asking if she should now tell their children the news about his cancer. Ross looked back at her as if he didn't understand what she wanted. Margaret sighed, took a deep breath, and began. They took the news better than expected. Margaret was surprised by this as well as by their lack of questions. Were they not even a little bit curious about their father's treatment? Ross seemed relieved that the conversation did not last long and went to the couch and turned on the television. Margaret felt slightly deflated as she cleared the table and put the leftovers in the fridge.

Both Nolan and Ruth were busy with their phones when Margaret returned to the den. She couldn't help herself from asking them why they were not more upset about the news.

"Mom, this happens to people when they get older," was Ruth's pragmatic reply.

Nolan added his opinion, "One of the guys at work got this and he said that if a man lives long enough, he'll get prostate cancer. I think he had radiation too and he didn't skip a beat. Worked through it and seemed just fine. Dad looks good too, but why is he having these injections you mentioned?"

"I don't really know why," Margaret replied, "The doctor just said he would have the injections every three months and I thought this is just the way the treatment is given. I guess I have to ask more questions."

Men with intermediate- or high-grade prostate cancer may have microscopic cancer cells that have the potential to cause spread in the body. Merely treating the prostate and adjacent tissues with radiation does not affect these microscopic cancer cells, but starving them of their fuel (testosterone) will limit their ability to grow and spread.

Ross had his first injection of Lupron before he started the radiation therapy. He didn't say much to Margaret about this, but when she asked, he showed her a small red patch of skin on his arm where the needle had been given.

"Did it hurt?" Margaret asked.

"Maybe a little bit, but wearing this tight sweater is making it uncomfortable and my boobs are so tender. Oh, I don't know how I am going to put up with all of this."

Margaret heard the start of panic in his voice. "Don't get ahead of yourself, Ross. You just had the injection today and you haven't had your usual nap. Why don't you lie down and I'll wake you a little later with a cup of hot cocoa?"

Ross smiled at her. She really was a great help to him, and he was buoyed by the thought of a nap with the promise of his favorite hot drink when he woke.

Within a few days, Ross started having hot flashes. He had never experienced anything like this before, and he was not happy. The feeling of heat came on suddenly, with barely any warning. One minute he was watching TV and the next he was sweating and pulling off his clothes. Margaret was sympathetic, but only to a point. She remembered the same thing happening to her when she was going through menopause, but as uncomfortable as she was, she never complained. Ross's reaction was a different story, of course. He made a huge fuss and woke her during the night when he had a hot flash; this annoyed her, but she also felt bad for him because this was not fun for him either. He was also more tired than usual, and this made things tense, because if he was not complaining or sweating profusely, he was sleeping!

Androgen deprivation therapy has a long list of side effects including hot flashes. These can be bothersome and often disrupt sleep and the man's partner as a result!

Ross insisted on going to his first radiation treatment alone. Margaret was annoyed but didn't say anything. This cancer of his was a real test of her patience and her ability to keep her thoughts to herself! He came home in good spirits and ate a large lunch, much to her surprise.

"It was a breeze!" he told her in response to her question about how the treatment had gone. "The therapists are great, and it was over and done in about fifteen minutes! I intend to finish as I have started—no problems at all!"

Margaret sent a private wish to the universe that this would be true, that he would not have any side effects and would sail through the weeks of treatment. But what she had read on Google gave her pause; it seemed that side effects were to be expected and some of them did not sound great at all! But overall, Ross seemed to be doing well. He went off to his radiation appointments without complaint and even seemed to look forward to seeing the therapists.

As the weeks went by, Ross grew more fatigued. Most afternoons, he had a nap in front of the TV and was grumpy when he woke up. Margaret expected this and tried to be as patient as she possibly could. It was not easy, however, and there were days when she wished she could go away somewhere and come back when his treatment was done. Ross was irritable and, at times, forgetful and this only made him more irritable. He was also more sensitive; one night he started to cry while watching the evening news. The final segment of the news was a story about a lost child who wandered into a forest and was found by a birdwatcher, cold and hungry, after three days. Ross was watching this with tears running down his cheeks, and Margaret was shocked—he was not one to cry easily, or at all! He seemed surprised that he was crying and quickly wiped his face with his sleeve. Margaret made a mental note to pay attention to his mood; she had experienced short bouts of depression over the years and was worried that his crying was a sign that he was depressed. She was highly sensitive to any signs of depression in herself and was worried about his crying.

Fatigue and increased emotional sensitivity are well known side effects of the lack of testosterone as a result of the hormone blockers. The emotional changes can be difficult to get used to, for both the man and his partner.

Eventually Ross completed his radiation therapy. Dr. Wong was surprised when he said that he had no side effects and Ross took this as a compliment, much to Margaret's irritation. Did he not remember how tired he was? When the doctor asked Ross how he was feeling on the androgen deprivation medication, he denied any side effects and said he was doing well. Margaret interrupted him and told the doctor that Ross was bothered by the hot flashes and that he was more irritable.

"Ah, yes," replied Dr. Wong, "That is not unusual. How bad are the hot flashes, Ross?"

"Um, not too bad I don't think."

"Ross, for goodness sake! Tell Dr. Wong the truth!" Margaret was furious at him for hiding the facts. "They are definitely bad! He's up a couple of times a night with them, and I have had to change the sheets on more than one occasion. All the tossing and turning keeps me up too!"

"Not getting good sleep can have an impact on mood, but there is not much we can do about the hot flashes. I could try you on some medication. Some men find that antidepressants help reduce the hot flashes. Are you interested in trying something?" Dr. Wong turned to his computer to create a prescription, but Margaret spoke up.

"I don't think he wants that, do you Ross? I read somewhere that there are other things we can do, like getting a fan in the bedroom. I'd rather we hold off on more medication."

"If that's okay with you, Ross, then I think that's a good place to start. We have some pamphlets about hot flashes and other side effects of the injections in the waiting room that you can pick up." Dr. Wong was once again looking at his computer monitor. "Anything else bothering you, Ross?"

Ross shook his head, but the doctor did not see this. Margaret took the silence as an opportunity to ask more questions.

"Dr. Wong? My husband is more moody than usual, and he seems to be more forgetful . . . I'm worried that it's, well . . . . dementia . . . I hate to say the word. Ross's father died of Alzheimer's."

Now Dr. Wong was looking at her. This concern was common, especially for the spouse of his patients. Dr. Wong tried to reassure her. "This is a source of anxiety for a lot of people. The association between the medication and dementia is not something we are sure of but there are many ongoing studies about this. From what we know at the present time, the medication may be associated with a decline in cognitive functioning, but the studies so far are not conclusive. And your husband has not been on the medication for very long, so I suspect that what you are seeing is not a sign of dementia."

Margaret tried to feel reassured, but she was still worried. She was not sure she had the patience to deal with her husband if he had dementia. She was struggling with him now!

Men may be more forgetful while on these medications and this raises concerns about dementia. However, there is no strong evidence that the medication is associated with the development of Alzheimer's and other forms of dementia.

"Anything else, Ross? Margaret?"

Dr. Wong looked like he wanted to end the appointment, so Margaret stood up and held out her hand to Ross. They thanked the doctor, who said that they would receive a letter with an appointment for his next injection. Ross fell asleep in the car going home, and Margaret welcomed the silence, as it gave her time to think. She decided that what she needed to do was keep a note of the side effects that Ross was experiencing.

Nothing much changed in the weeks after the completion of his radiation therapy. Ross napped most days after lunch, and this gave Margaret some alone time that she often used to go for a walk around the neighborhood. Ross usually declined her offer to walk with her, so she went off by herself while he slept. One afternoon she insisted that he come with her; in the front yard of a house two blocks away was the most magnificent display of dahlias. She loved these flowers with their heavy heads and perfectly formed petals, but had never had any success growing them.

Ross agreed reluctantly and went to their bedroom to change into walking clothes. When he didn't return, Margaret grew worried. What was holding him up? She walked to their bedroom, calling his name. She was shocked to see him sitting on the bed, clothes strewn on the bed and at his feet.

"What is it! Are you okay? Why are you just sitting there?" Margaret tried to not panic but she was confused. He looked okay, so why was he just sitting there and why were there clothes all over the room? "What is wrong, Ross? Talk to me!"

Ross didn't say anything and pointed to his abdomen. Margaret looked where he was pointing but didn't see what was upsetting him.

"Ross, use your words, please! What is it? Are you in pain? Did you hurt yourself?"

"Can't you see?" Ross was yelling, "Nothing fits! Look at this T-shirt! It's too tight and I look stupid!"

Margaret looked at her husband again. His T-shirt was stretched tightly over his stomach and about an inch of skin was showing between the T-shirt and his pants. She realized that she had not really looked at him for a while and his stomach was larger than it had ever been. How had she not noticed that he had gained weight?

Weight gain, especially in the abdominal area, is a common complaint of men on androgen deprivation therapy. Loss of upper body muscle strength often occurs as well, and there is a risk for loss of bone density with long-term use of these medications.

There was no walk for them that afternoon. Ross was in a foul mood and left Margaret to tidy their bedroom. This annoyed her, and they avoided each other for the rest of the day. Ruth called to ask if she could stop by before dinner, but Margaret told her that they were busy. She felt bad about lying to their daughter, but the frosty atmosphere would only prompt questions and Margaret did not know what she would say. Later that evening, she sat down next to her husband while he watched

TV and tried to hold his hand. He pulled away quite forcefully and stomped off to their bedroom.

What was that about? Margaret had not anticipated that he would storm off, and she sat on the couch for a while, trying to figure out what was going on. While his response to her trying to hold his hand was unexpected, she realized that they had not touched each other, not even a kiss on the cheek, for weeks! She remembered Dr. Wong saying something about sexual changes with the medication, but she had not really listened as there was so much information to take in. At the time, sex was not a priority, although it had been important throughout most of their marriage. Make-up sex was what probably saved them from divorce so many times. That's how they resolved their fights, and of course things had changed over the years, and sex was not the same, but this was an important part of how they related to one another!

She looked on the internet for information about the sexual side effects of the medication, and there was a lot! Over and over, she read the same thing—men on androgen deprivation therapy lost their desire for sex and stopped having erections. Why had she not known this? Was this why he pulled away from her or was it something else? She decided that she needed another test to try to figure this out.

The opportunity came the next evening. They had not talked much over the course of the day, but this was not unusual. Ross opened a bottle of wine with dinner and chatted with her as if nothing had happened the previous night, and it felt like they were back on track. Margaret took a deep breath and walked up to Ross, who was putting the dishes in the sink. She put her arms around him from behind and he twisted away from her, almost falling.

"What are you doing?" His voice was angry.

"I'm, I'm . . . I just want to hug you! Is that a crime?" Margaret was about to cry, and she tried to swallow her words, knowing that if she said any more, she would be sobbing and Ross hated that.

Ross glared at her, the expression on his face was one that Margaret had never seen before. Why was he so angry? What was happening?

Margaret didn't get much sleep that night. Ross didn't come to bed and she heard him tossing and turning on the couch. She thought about going to him, but then she remembered the look on his face when she had tried to hug him. She eventually dozed off close to 5 a.m. and woke when the sunlight streamed through a gap in the curtains. She lay in bed for a few minutes, the events of the night before entering her memory like an old film reel. She had to do something about this, so she got up, showered quickly, and called Dr. Wong's office at exactly 9 a.m. when they opened.

The receptionist was helpful even though Dr. Wong wasn't in yet. Margaret told her that she wanted the name of a counselor; she didn't say why and the receptionist did not ask for any information and gave her the name of someone whose office was in the same building. Before she lost her nerve, Margaret called this person's office. There was a voice message that said that Dr. Ronson would call back within twenty-four hours.

"So now I wait," thought Margaret, as she went to look for Ross. She found him sitting on the deck, a mug of coffee on the table in front of him. His hair was messy, and he was wearing the clothes he had on from the previous day.

"You okay?" he asked her without looking up.

"Sure, you?" Margaret did not feel okay, but she was not sure how to respond. She didn't know if she should tell him that she had called Dr. Wong's office. She was afraid that he would be angry, and she was too tired to get into a fight with him. As she went back into the house get pour herself some coffee, her phone rang. It was Dr. Ronson's office, so she hurried into the bedroom to take the call. To her surprise, it was Dr. Ronson, herself, who had called her back. She sounded businesslike, but she had a kind voice and within minutes, Margaret had an appointment for the next week.

She was nervous as she drove to the appointment even though she had looked forward to meeting with Dr. Ronson. She and Ross had not talked about what had happened and had kept any conversation superficial. She arrived a full ten minutes early and sat on a chair outside the office until the door opened, exactly at her appointment time. The young woman who invited her in introduced herself as Dr. Ronson. She explained that she was a psychologist who specialized in treating people with any kind of illness. Her office was small with colorful pictures on the walls and a set of leather furniture, a couch for patients and a chair for the psychologist.

"What brings you in today? Is it okay if I call you Margaret?"

Margaret nodded. She opened her mouth to speak but instead burst into tears. Dr. Ronson passed her a box of tissues and waited while

Margaret stopped crying, wiped her face and blew her nose. She took a deep breath, sighed, and then told the psychologist what had happened. She talked without interruption for almost ten minutes, barely stopping to breathe, her eyes focused on her lap. When she stopped, she sighed again and looked at Dr. Ronson.

"Would you believe I have heard a similar story from many different women?" the psychologist asked gently. "What you describe is so common in couples where the man is on this hormone therapy. What seems to be happening is that, in the absence of testosterone, his desire or libido vanishes, and he stops any kind of physical contact with his partner. When his partner tries to touch him, even in a nonsexual way, the man reacts negatively, perhaps thinking that the woman in this instance, is initiating sex. Because the medication also causes erectile dysfunction, he feels threatened or sad that he cannot respond and so rejects any touch. This can cause a lot of hurt feelings and misunderstandings, and of course a lot of distress for both . . ."

"Oh, that makes sense." Margaret was shocked that she had not realized what was going in Ross's mind. She had so many questions about this, and Dr. Ronson had the answers to all of them, and before she knew it, Dr. Ronson was telling her that their time was up. The hour had flown by, and she felt so much more informed by their conversation.

Testosterone plays an important role in male desire and sexual function, and most men will experience a decrease in both sexual interest and erectile function while on androgen deprivation therapy.

"Do you think your husband would be willing to come in with you to talk about this?" Dr. Ronson had a smile on her face; it was obvious that she had asked this question many times before.

"I'm not sure. He doesn't even know I'm here."

"I understand, but if you are not on the same page, you may not find a way through this. I know that men don't like to talk about sex or feelings, or at least they don't find it easy to talk about this in a serious way. It's easier to joke or pretend that nothing's wrong."

"You're right, Dr. Ronson. I'll talk to him but I'm not confident he'll agree."

Margaret left the psychologist's office with more understanding and the smallest flutter of hope in her heart. Now she just had to persuade Ross that they needed to talk about this, and it would be good if they could do that with Dr. Ronson.

CONCLUSION

Androgen deprivation therapy lowers testosterone to very low levels; the medication is prescribed for men who have radiation therapy in certain instances as well as for those with advanced or recurrent prostate cancer. The medication has many side effects that impact sexual function, body image, bone and cardiovascular health, and potentially cognitive function as well. As with many other treatments for prostate cancer, there is an impact on the partner of the man as well. Accurate and timely information about what to expect when the man is on this treatment is vital for the couple.

Reflective Questions

After reading this chapter:

- How can a partner/spouse seek their own support when the man is reluctant to tell other family members about their cancer diagnosis?
- What changes might you expect in your own relationship if your spouse experiences any/all of the side effects of androgen therapy?
- How would you prepare to deal with the impact of these changes on your relationship?

Chapter Nine

Clinical Trials
He'd Like to Enroll

Participating in a clinical trial is an altruistic endeavor that many men with prostate undertake in order to find new treatments or interventions. This chapter will describe the process of taking part in a study of a new treatment or medication through the story of a couple who have some misunderstandings about what it means to be a participant in a study.

Samuel Harris, an African American man, is seventy-one years old and has a long history of prostate cancer. He was first diagnosed at the age of sixty-seven with unfavorable intermediate-risk disease and chose brachytherapy, a form of radiation, as treatment. His PSA went down to 2 but then started to rise. His radiation oncologist prescribed androgen deprivation therapy and, initially, this lowered his PSA to 0.5, but then it started to rise again. Late last year a lesion was found on his bone scan, meaning that he now had metastatic disease. He was referred to a medical oncologist, Dr. Sanders, who worked out of a well-known cancer center an hour's drive from their home. Dr. Sanders added a new medication in addition to the testosterone-lowering injections, and Samuel was hopeful that this one would work. But his PSA kept rising.

African American men have the highest rates of new prostate cancer diagnoses and the highest death rates from this cancer, compared to men of other races. Prostate cancer that has spread outside the prostate is called metastatic disease. The first line of treatment for this is androgen deprivation, which deprives the cancer of its fuel, testosterone, as you read in the previous chapter.

Samuel's wife, Bertha, was not aware of the details of any of this. She was two years older than him and avoided medical care as much as she could. She had never shown any interest in going to appointments with him and she showed no curiosity about his diagnosis or treatment. In the beginning this had hurt his feelings and, as a result, he did not share his concerns with her. When he thought about it, he was sad, because going through the treatment alone was not easy, but after fifty-one years of marriage, he knew he couldn't change her. They had no children and no family close to them, but Samuel had friends, a group of African American men, who played chess together, and he depended on them for advice. Of the six men, three had been diagnosed with prostate cancer over the years.

Every morning they sat under the trees in the park, their chairs arranged around collapsible tables that Jacob, the unofficial leader of the group, brought with him to their chess games. There were only three of them that day; this suited Samuel as he wanted to talk about something and one of the three who were missing often made jokes, and he was in no mood for humor.

"Gentlemen, if I may, I have a question . . ." Samuel's tone was serious and the other two men looked up at him. "So . . . Jacob and Miles, this is really for you . . . you have walked the walk, same as me . . . but my PSA is going up again, even though I have been taking that new stuff the doc ordered for me. I don't know what to do now." Samuel was looking at his hands that were clasped on the table. His shoulders were slumped, and he sounded dejected.

Jacob cleared his throat; he needed time to craft a response. "Well, my friend, I don't rightly know. I'm just an old man with old man problems, same as the rest of us."

Miles looked like someone had hit him over the head. He usually had a lot to say, but in the moment, he was speechless. He and Jacob looked at each other; they had both had surgery, Jacob last year and Miles ten years ago. Their PSA values had remained consistently low, in the undetectable range, and for this they were grateful. Seeing Samuel like this, the worry reflected in his posture, made them upset. They used to compare their PSA results, but since Samuel's numbers kept going in the wrong direction, they were careful talking about their appointments with their doctors.

"What does your wife say?" This was the best that Miles could contribute in the moment and he immediately regretted his words.

Samuel's eyes had filled with tears. "She's not interested . . . not in my health and not in hers. She says that if I just ate properly, fruits and vegetables, you know, rabbit food I call it, this wouldn't have happened. I haven't told her about this, and she doesn't ask."

Jacob tried to steer the conversation away from talk about Samuel's wife. She was an odd one in his opinion. She kept to herself, had not been interested in meeting his own wife, his beloved Sheila, who had passed away from breast cancer six months ago. Jacob knew that no amount of fruits or vegetables could cure cancer. If it could, he would have planted a garden to keep his Sheila alive. "But what does your doctor say?"

Samuel sighed. He had another appointment with Dr. Sanders at the beginning of the next month, and he wanted to go to that with some idea of what he might say. "My doc, Dr. Sanders, said he would give me some more information when I see him next month. I just don't know."

Miles was hesitant to voice an opinion. Unlike Jacob, his treatment was years ago, and he didn't think about having cancer at all. He didn't have any doctor's appointments anymore, at least not with the surgeon who had taken his prostate out. He had other problems now, his blood pressure was high and he had put on some weight over the past years. His wife baked every weekend for church and he loved her cookies so much and could not stop sneaking one, or three, when they came out of the oven. "Maybe you don't need to know anything until you talk to him."

"Yeah," Jacob agreed, "Maybe Miles is right. Wait and see what your doctor says and then make a decision."

Samuel shrugged. It was so difficult dealing with this, and he needed all the support he could get. But Miles was right; he was jumping the gun and needed to wait until he saw Dr. Sanders. "Are we going to get to any chess today?" he asked the other two men, his voice too loud. And so, two of them started the game while the other watched.

The day of his appointment arrived in what seemed like the blink of an eye. This is how things went when you're old, he thought to himself, the days, weeks, and months coming at once, like a fast-moving train. He dressed in his church clothes, a suit and tie with shiny shoes, to show the doctor respect. The wait seemed hours long because he kept checking his watch. He had arrived at the cancer clinic almost forty-five minutes early, so he needed to exercise some patience.

He was shown into one of the examination rooms by the receptionist. He was usually told to undress and put on one of the blue paper gowns, but this time she told him to take a seat and not to change his clothes. What did that mean?

He didn't have to wait long to find out. Within just a few minutes there was a knock on the door and Dr. Sanders entered, followed by a young woman holding his chart.

"Hello there, Samuel!" Dr. Sanders seemed cheerful, "Let me introduce you to Anita, one of the clinical trial nurses here."

The young woman reached over to shake his hand, almost dropping the chart that she held. "Please to meet you, Samuel. Is it okay if I use your first name?" She seemed flustered and blushed, her freckles darkening.

"That's fine, Miss . . . may I call you Anita?" Samuel was old-fashioned that way.

"Of course, sir." Anita's face grew even more red.

"Okay, let's get this started," Dr. Sanders took over from them. "Samuel, as you are aware, your PSA has continued to rise despite the new medication we put you on . . ."

Samuel interrupted him. "Excuse me, Doc, but what is my PSA now?"

"Hmmm," Dr. Sanders took the chart from Anita. "It's up to 13. That's quite a jump from where it was when we started you on the additional medication. Are you having any pain?"

Samuel shook his head. He was worried about what the doctor had told him about the spot they saw on the bone scan, but he felt fine other than the fatigue from the medication.

"I want to talk to you about being part of a clinical trial of a new drug. That's why I brought Anita with me. I'm going to leave you with her to explain the study. Anita, take it away."

And with that, Dr. Sanders left the room.

A clinical trial tests whether a new treatment is safe
and effective and also better than the currently available treatment. The treatment may be a new chemotherapy drug, a new kind of radiation therapy, or new
way of giving medication or radiation.

Anita spoke to Samuel for close to twenty minutes. She talked slowly
and stopped frequently to see if he had any questions. Samuel found it
difficult to concentrate on what she was saying, despite how carefully
she explained everything. She used lots of numbers and words that he
didn't understand, and he was embarrassed to ask questions, so he sat
quietly, nodding his head. To his relief, she eventually stopped talking.

"Samuel, I know that was a lot of information and I have some pamphlets that explain the trial in more detail that you can take home and
talk with your family about this."

Samuel sighed. Who was he supposed to talk to? Bertha was not interested in anything to do with his cancer, and he was confused. "Miss,
to be honest, I don't know what to do. What do I get out of this?"

"That's a good question, sir."

Depending on the nature of the trial, taking part may
be a purely altruistic act; future people with the same
disease will benefit. For others, participation means
they will get a new treatment that may benefit them.

"Okay, I understand that . . . but will I get the new treatment?" Samuel
was still confused, and he was scared that perhaps he would not get any
treatment at all. He wanted to talk to Dr. Sanders about this, but when
he asked this lady if she could get the doctor to come back, she told him
that it was not possible. Samuel did not understand why he couldn't talk
to his doctor; now he was tired and thirsty, and he wanted to go home.
"Okay, then I'll do it. Will you tell Dr. Sanders that I'll do whatever he
wants me to do?"

"Hang on a minute, sir," Anita was concerned that Samuel was not making an informed decision about participating in the study. "I think we need to talk about this a bit more."

"What's there to talk about?" Samuel was growing more annoyed by the minute; he felt like she was treating him as if he were stupid and he did not like that at all.

Anita took a deep breath. "Okay, I'll see if I can find Dr. Sanders. Can I get you something to drink while you wait?"

Samuel grunted. Maybe some water would help.

> Many people agree to take part in a study to help others and for personal hope (Dellson et al. 2018). The main barrier to participation is not being offered the chance to take part.

Samuel sat alone for quite a while after Anita brought him a bottle of water. He wasn't sure why Dr. Sanders had not talked to him directly in the first place, and he wanted to hear the doctor's opinion about all of this. It seemed to Samuel that his doctor was in favor of this, so why didn't he explain things to him?

After what seemed like hours, but was closer to twenty minutes, Dr. Sanders came back with Anita close behind. "Anita tells me that you wanted to talk to me." Dr. Sanders seemed rushed; he didn't sit down, and his hands were in the pockets of his white coat.

"Yes I did, sir! I want to know what you think about this study or whatever! You're my doctor and I want to know your opinion!"

"It's my job to tell patients when there is a trial that they are eligible for. I have to maintain distance from giving the patient information because I am involved in the study, and I don't want you to feel pressured to participate. That is why Anita is here, to tell you about the trial and answer any questions. Now I have to go back to my clinic. Anita will remain to answer any questions you may have."

Samuel was disappointed with Dr. Sanders's response. He did not know what to do, and the doctor had not been any help. He was frustrated and tired, and he wanted to go home.

When the treating physician recommends that a patient take part in a trial, this can be seen as coercive because the patient may think that if he doesn't agree, his care will be affected negatively.

Anita sat down on a chair next to Samuel and handed him a binder with multiple sheets of paper that were organized into sections. He felt nervous just looking at what she had handed him. What was he supposed to do with this?

"This is the material about the study, Samuel. There is a lot of information that you should know, and before you agree to be part of the clinical trial, you need to read this, and then I can answer any questions you have, and then finally you can agree to be part of this, or not. I don't want you to feel any pressure from me or Dr. Sanders. Your decision is okay with us either way."

"But if Dr. Sanders thinks that this is the right thing for me to do, then maybe I should just agree." Samuel's voice was uncertain as he stared first at the binder in his lap and then at Anita.

"Is there someone that you can talk to about this? A family member or a friend?"

Samuel shook his head. Bertha would not help, and he didn't want to bother his friends.

Anita's voice was gentle as she looked him in the eyes. "You can take the binder home and read the material in there. Take as long as you need and call me if you have any questions. My phone number is on the first page."

Samuel stood up, the binder clasped in his hands. "Thank you, Miss. I'm sorry."

Anita smiled at him as he turned and walked away. Her heart ached for this man, one of many she saw who struggled with the complex task of agreeing to be part of a study. She knew that the material and consent form were complicated and difficult to read for some, but anyone agreeing to participate needed to understand exactly what they were agreeing to.

Health literacy refers to the ability of a person to access, read, and understand basic health information needed to make decisions about their health (Kieffer Campbell 2020). Even people who have a good education may have difficulty understanding information about their health; the information they receive may be very technical and in "medical language" that is not familiar to them.

Samuel went home with the binder on the seat next to him; it felt like another presence in the car, and while he tried to ignore it, he was aware that it was lying there, waiting for him to read the pages. He put the binder on the kitchen table and made himself a cup of coffee. Bertha looked at it as she walked to the fridge but didn't ask him about it. He thought about telling her what it was and even asking if she wanted to know more, but he was afraid that if she declined, his feelings would be hurt once again.

When his coffee was ready, he sat down at the table and started reading. Bertha glanced at him but didn't say anything. He tried to get her attention by sighing and ruffling the pages, but she walked out of the room, taking a bite out of the peach she had taken from the fridge. He felt so alone and put the binder down, open at the first page where Anita's phone number was printed.

The next morning, he tried again, turning the pages over and reading, his lips moving silently. He understood some of it, and when he got to parts that looked like a foreign language, he skipped to the next part. Eventually, he got to the end of the pages. He was still not 100 percent sure of the details, but he understood that he would be getting some new medication, and this made him happy. What he was taking now did not seem to be working, so this was a chance to make things better. He found a pen next to the telephone, took a deep breath, and signed the page that said he was willing to be part of the study.

It was still early, but he took a chance and called Anita. She didn't answer so he left her a voice message. "Hello, hello? Anita? This is

Samuel. I'm going to do it. I mean I signed the form. So now what do I do?

He felt lighter now that he had signed the form and he hoped that Dr. Sanders would be pleased with him. Now that he had made the decision, he wanted to tell someone about this. He was glad that he was going to meet with his friends at their regular chess date and he dressed quickly. He left the house without saying good-bye to Bertha, who was in the back yard tending to her tomato plants.

He waited for the others to arrive. It was a beautiful day and he sat on a bench, his face turned to the sun. Jacob and Miles arrived together; they lived close to one another and had known each other for more than thirty years when they first started working for the city. The others, John, Edward and James, arrived shortly after them. Miles had set up the chessboards and the men settled down to play. Samuel hung back until the others had paired off and then he took the chair opposite Miles.

"Hey, Miles, can we talk about something? I need to tell someone and well, you've walked the walk with this cancer thing."

"Sure thing, Brother Samuel, what's happening?" Miles leaned forward, the chess board ignored for the moment. Samuel told him about the study that he had agreed to join. His brief description sounded hopeful and Miles hesitated before saying anything. Samuel was looking at him, waiting to hear what he thought. "Brother Samuel, my friend . . . do you trust these people?'

Samuel was taken aback; this is not what he expected Miles' response to be. "Um, why wouldn't I trust them? He's my doctor, and of course I trust him! Why would he want to do wrong by me?"

Miles took a deep breath, thinking how he was going to explain what he was thinking. "Do you know about Tuskegee? Do you know what they did to our people?" As much as he tried, Miles could not keep his voice down.

"No, what's this you speak of? Who did what to our people?"

The other men were now paying attention, but Miles ignored them. He was shocked that Samuel did not know about what had happened way back when, but he tried to not let his friend notice his disbelief.

Starting in 1932, six hundred poor, Black sharecroppers in Macon County, Alabama, were enrolled in a
long-term study of progression in men with syphilis.
The men were not treated and, instead, were observed
to see if the disease progressed differently in Black
men than in White men. The study continued until
1972, and many died from complications of the disease, and many of their female partners and babies
were infected. (Sacks 2021)

The men were quiet after Miles described how the study of the sharecroppers had influenced how some Black people viewed research and
their lack of trust in the health care system. The other men had heard
about this before, but Samuel had not. As he thought about what Miles
had described, he wondered if that was why Bertha ignored her own
health care. He wanted to talk to her about that, and maybe that would
open the door to a conversation with her about his illness.

No one wanted to play chess after that; they were silent as they
packed up the tables and chess sets. Miles offered to accompany Samuel to his home, but Samuel assured him that was not necessary. They
separated at the entrance to the park, hugging each other instead of their
usual fist bumps. They all had a lot to think about.

When Samuel got home, he found Bertha in the garden. He started to
ask her if she knew about the Tuskegee study and if this was the reason
that she did not go to the doctor but he was interrupted by the sound of
the telephone ringing. He went inside and answered the phone.

"Hello. This is the Harris residence."

"Samuel, Mr. Harris, this is Anita. How are you? I got your message
and I am so happy to hear that you have signed the consent form. I'd
like to set up a time for you to come in to get some tests done before
you start the medication."

Samuel was not sure what to say next. Yes, he had signed the form,
but he did not know about that awful thing that happened to his people.
He took a deep breath. "Miss, I heard something today that has me
turned around and I'm not sure that I want to be a guinea pig for you
folks."

Anita hesitated before answering. She suspected that she knew the reason for his change of mind, but she knew that she had to listen before talking. "Mr. Harris? What did you hear?"

Samuel told her what Miles had said. His voice was loud and he felt himself getting angry at her even though he knew that what happened was not her fault.

"I can hear how deeply this has affected you, sir," she said quietly, "The consent form you signed, and the details in there about the study, is a direct response to what happened to those men. We can never let something like that happen again."

Samuel grunted; he was not sure what to do.

"Mr. Harris, this study may give you a chance to receive a treatment that can help you. If you get the experimental treatment, this may be of benefit to you."

"What do you mean when you say that *if* I get the new treatment?" Samuel was confused by what Anita had said. He thought that by taking part in the study he would get the medication that would control his cancer.

"The study compares the treatment you are on now with the new experimental medication. The consent form you signed talks about that in detail, Mr. Harris. You will be randomized to either receiving the medication you are on now, or the addition of the new medication. I'm sorry that you did not realize this."

"What do you mean by randomized?" Samuel was confused; he did not remember reading anything about this. But to be honest, he didn't really read all the pages before signing his name.

"Okay, let me explain what randomization means . . ."

Randomization means that every person in the trial has an equal chance of getting the new treatment or not. It can be compared to flipping a coin—heads or tails—and that determines which group you fall into for the trial.

"I have to think about this, Miss," replied Samuel. He was still confused, but one thing he did know what that he didn't want to be in the group that did not get the new medication.

"That's fine, Mr. Harris. If you want, we can meet again for me to go through the consent form and the details of the study. Would you like to bring a member of your family with you?"

There was silence but Anita could hear Samuel breathing. "How about you come in later this afternoon or tomorrow morning if that is better for you?"

"Um, let's do it tomorrow if that's okay."

Anita agreed and asked him to come in at 11 a.m. Samuel ended the call and went out to the garden. He wanted his wife to know what he had been offered, and he wanted—no he knew—that he needed her support. She was inspecting her tomato plants but listened as he told her about the study and what Miles had told him. He needed to repeat the story of the Tuskegee sharecroppers; the injustice brought tears to her eyes. When Samuel told her that he was thinking about being in a study, her response was immediate.

"What happens if you don't do this?"

"I guess things will get worse for me. Dr. Sanders said that the injections and pills I am getting now aren't working anymore."

"Then you must do it! You must try this!"

Samuel was surprised at her response. She had never shown any interest in his treatment and he hadn't told her that his PSA was rising. But here she was, encouraging him to take part in the study. Maybe she cared after all."

Encouragement from family and friends may play a role in a man's decision to take part in a clinical trial. Family members may be desperate to keep the man with them under any circumstances and they think that a clinical trial offers hope for that.

Samuel hesitated before asking Bertha to go with him to the appointment with Anita. "I have an appointment tomorrow with the lady who is involved in the study. Do you want to come with me?"

"Do you want me to?"

"Yes, of course I do! I want you to be by my side, I always have! But you seemed not interested." Samuel's voice cracked, and he felt tears coming to his eyes.

"Okay then. I'll come with you. No need to get upset about it!" Bertha turned back to her tomato plants and Samuel stood looking at her back. He was not sure what or why she suddenly seemed interested, but he would take this as a good sign.

There are resources available to help you understand the processes involved in taking part in clinical trials as well as what trials are available and open to recruitment (see chapter 1).

Bertha was a woman of her word. She went with him to the appointment and asked good questions that he had not thought of. In fact, he had hardly asked any questions and he was embarrassed about that. It was wonderful having Bertha by his side; he was not sure why she had changed her mind, but he was glad that she was there. Her support of the study helped him make his decision. He handed over the signed copy of the consent form, this time sure that he wanted to do this.

CONCLUSION

Taking part in a clinical trial or study is a personal choice. The study may not benefit the man, himself, but will provide information about whether the new treatment is effective for other men when the study is over. There are clear guidelines that all studies need to adhere to; these protect participants in research. The most important of these is the need for informed consent that relies on the person being told and understanding all the details of the study before agreeing to participate. Family members need to know these details, as well, so that they can provide support for the man as he decides whether to participate or not.

Reflective Questions

After reading this chapter:

- What do you understand about the reasons that a man would want to take part in a clinical trial?

- Why is participation in a clinical trial a voluntary action?
- What would you tell your partner if he is unsure of taking part in a clinical trial?
- What are the reasons that you and other family members should also be informed about the study?

REFERENCES

Dellson, P., K. Nilsson, H. Jernström, and C. Carlsson. 2018. "Patients' reasoning regarding the decision to participate in clinical cancer trials: An interview study." *Trials* 19 (1): 528. doi: 10.1186/s13063-018-2916-9.

Kieffer Campbell, J. 2020. "Health literacy in adult oncology: An integrative review." *Oncology Nursing Forum* 47 (1): 18–32. doi: 10.1188/20.onf.18 -32.

Sacks, T., K. Savin, Q. Walton. 2021. "How ancestral trauma informs patients' health decision making." *AMA Journal of Ethics* 23 (2): e183–88. doi: 10.1001/amajethics.2021.183.

Chapter Ten

The Role of
Communication in Relationships

"How Can We Talk about This?"

Communication is central to working together after a diagnosis and treatment for prostate cancer. But couples often don't communicate effectively; they buffer to protect each other's feelings and may make assumptions about what the other person is thinking and feeling. This may lead to confusion and conflict, as well as hurt feelings and unnecessary fears. This chapter highlights the story of a couple who have been married for ten years but find themselves having difficulty understanding each other's perspectives. They ultimately agree to seeing a counselor who supports them in finding more effective communication strategies.

Al and Pauline have been married for ten years; it's a second marriage for them both after their first marriages ended in divorce years ago. They are both fifty-five years old. Pauline has one daughter from her first marriage. Al never had children. He was treated for lymphoma in his early twenties, and the chemotherapy made him infertile; he blames this for the end of his first marriage, because his ex-wife wanted children. He fell in love with Pauline on a blind date set up by friends, but she was not sure she was interested in another relationship after her divorce. Her friends had pressured her to meet Al, and ten years later, here they were, facing a challenge that neither thought would happen. Wasn't having cancer once enough for Al?

Al was diagnosed with localized, low-risk prostate cancer almost a year ago. Within weeks, he had surgery to remove his prostate despite Pauline's encouraging him to wait before making a treatment decision.

189

On one hand, she understood why he was in a hurry to get treatment but, on the other hand, she thought he was not taking enough time to make sure that he needed the surgery immediately. But what was done was done, and they moved forward. Al recovered well; at fifty-five years of age, he was healthy and physically fit. He cycled to work every day, a distance of eight miles, no matter how bad the weather. As the manager of a bookstore, he spent most of the day sitting, and he enjoyed his daily commute on wheels. Despite her misgivings about the surgery, Pauline was pleasantly surprised by how soon he was back on his bicycle. She had been afraid that the surgery would affect his daily activities, but after just a month, he had gone back to work and their life seemed the same as it was before.

At his six-week appointment with the surgeon, Al was pleased to hear that the cancer was confirmed to be localized to the prostate and the lymph nodes were clear. He called Pauline as soon as he left the doctor's office.

"It's all good, honey! Dr. Trent was really pleased with my recovery and I only need to see him in three months! I think I'm going to go to work. I'll see you close to six, okay?

Pauline was relieved that the cancer had not spread, but why was he rushing to work today? She had arranged to have the afternoon off from work so that she could be with him after his appointment, just in case the news was not good, and now she would have to spend the afternoon alone.

"I was just about to leave work to come home."

She tried to not sound disappointed. "No need, Paul."

Al had started abbreviating her name soon after they started dating. She didn't really like it but had never said anything to him. In the beginning of their relationship, she didn't want to hurt his feelings and, as time went by, she got used to it. When she thought about it, she realized that she spent a lot of time doing what he wanted rather than what she wanted, and this made her feel a mixture of sadness and anger. But it was too late to change this; ten years was a long time, in her mind, and she didn't want to rock the boat. She had been outspoken in her first marriage and look what happened! Divorced at twenty-five years old with a five-year old daughter to support. Her first husband had not provided any financial support after the divorce, and she had struggled to provide for the two of them. The twenty years she had spent without a partner were hard, and she was determined to work on her marriage to Al; if that meant not upsetting him about anything, then that is what she would do.

Al came home just after 6 p.m. and acted as if nothing had happened. Pauline was ready to celebrate; she had prepared a delicious dinner for him in case the news from his doctor was not good and he needed comforting. She was happy that now the meal would be for a celebration. She had set the table with the good china, but he hardly seemed to notice. He ate the roast chicken with potatoes and mushrooms as if this were a regular dinner. Pauline felt herself getting more and more resentful, but she said nothing.

Over the next months. she continued to say nothing as he grew more and more quiet and withdrawn. He had never been one to share his feelings and this had never really bothered her until now. She wanted to know how he was doing, not just physically but more importantly emotionally, but he kept his feelings to himself. She didn't say anything when he started going to work earlier and earlier, missing what used to be their usual first coffee of the day at the kitchen counter. It had been their habit to each take part of the daily newspaper, interrupting the silence with a comment about something they had read that would be of interest to the other. Now he was gone before her alarm went off. He didn't text her during the day, as he normally would, and he came home later and later. Daylight saving time had ended almost two weeks before and he didn't seem to mind coming home in the dark. She worried about him on his bike in the dark; he usually wore a fluorescent vest when he rode to and from work, but she found it in the garage, hanging behind the door under an abandoned raincoat. Her worry turned to fear. What was happening?

She tried talking to him one night after dinner. He had hardly eaten what was on his plate and, as she cleared the table, she realized that this was now a pattern. If he served himself, he put small amounts of food on his plate and, even then, he left some behind. If she plated his dinner, he ate just enough for her to see that he had tried everything, but most of his dinner ended up in the garbage. She turned back to look at him and she was shocked to see that he had lost weight. He had never been overweight, but now there was a big gap between his shirt collar and his neck, and his face looked drawn.

"Honey, Al, what's going on? What are you feeling? I'm worried about you." Her voice had an edge of desperation and as the words left her mouth, she saw him start to rise from his chair.

"There is NOTHING wrong with me, Pauline! Just leave me alone!" And with that he walked out of the kitchen, his chair almost tipping over.

When the man withdraws from his partner, this should be a red flag in the relationship. How the partner responds will influence how long the situation continues. Avoiding talking about what has changed makes the problem bigger as the days go by.

One morning, Pauline came down to the kitchen to have her coffee before going to work at the community college where she was the assistant to the admissions director. She was surprised to see that Al was still there. She had gotten used to his absence in the mornings and, without thinking, she put her arms around him from behind, just as she used to do in the "before" times. His reaction shocked her. He jumped up as if she had punched him; the chair fell over, hitting her leg as it fell to the floor. He didn't say anything as he pushed past her, heading to the kitchen door.

Pauline stood, the back of the chair resting on her left foot. Her hands were shaking as she searched on her phone for the number for the student health clinic at the college where she worked. She needed to talk to someone about what was happening; she couldn't tell any of her friends because that would influence how they related to Al and that felt like a betrayal. She had a good relationship with the nurse practitioner who worked part-time at the student health clinic. Staff were also allowed to use the clinic for their health care, and she regarded this as one of the most important aspects of her employment.

The receptionist at the clinic must have heard something in Pauline's voice because, after a brief hold, she told Pauline to come in at noon that afternoon. Pauline was grateful, but she also felt a little guilty because that was the nurse practitioner's lunch break. However, her guilty feelings did not prevent her from accepting the last-minute appointment. She drove to work and parked in her usual spot, hardly recalling how she got there. For the rest of the morning, she was distracted; emails were ignored and she let most of the phone calls go to voice mail. Fortunately, her boss was at on out-of-town meeting that day, and she watched the minutes tick by. She left her office thirty minutes before her appointment time and wandered around the bookstore until it was time for her to see the nurse practitioner.

The nursing assistant escorted her to the nurse practitioner's office. Pauline had been a patient of Lisa's, the nurse practitioner, since she first started her practice at the student health clinic. Five years ago, Lisa had seemed to lack confidence, but Pauline found that she really liked the young woman. When she didn't have an answer to a question, she was honest in saying so and always contacted Pauline when she found one. She was easy to talk to and did not book ten-minute appointments like the physicians at the clinic. Lisa was sitting at her desk, a half-eaten sandwich beside her.

"I'm so sorry to disturb your lunch hour." Pauline began apologizing before Lisa had said a word.

"Oh, don't worry, I usually eat at my desk while I catch up on the morning's charting. I'll always make time for you, Pauline, you know that. You were my first staff person I had as a patient here at the college and I was terrified that I would mess up."

Pauline started to laugh at the comment, but her laughter turned to tears.

"What's wrong? What's going on, Pauline?"

Pauline wiped the tears from her face with the back of her hand, ignoring the box of tissues that Lisa offered. She shook her head, sighed and started to tell Lisa what was happening at home. Lisa knew that Pauline's husband had been diagnosed with prostate cancer and had undergone surgery, but she had not seen Pauline since then. She listened to Pauline's description of how her husband's behavior had changed over the past months. Her mug of coffee sat untouched next to her keyboard and her eyes never left Pauline's face.

"What do you think is going on with your husband?" Lisa was always careful to ask her patients what they thought before offering an opinion or advice. She had learned through experience that most people only asked for help after they had tried to figure things out for themselves.

"I don't know . . . it feels like he's checked out of our marriage." Pauline paused as she thought about Al's behavior and then her face took on an expression of horror. "Do you think he's . . . he's having an affair?" Tears were running down her cheeks again and this time she took a tissue out of the box that Lisa had placed on the arm of the chair where she was sitting.

"It may not be that he's having an affair," Lisa reassured her patient, "But from what you have described, he may be depressed."

Pauline looked at Lisa with a confused expression on her face. "Depressed? He's never been depressed before. It's not something I ever thought he would be."

Men who are diagnosed with prostate cancer report depression, starting at the time of diagnosis (Sefik et al. 2020). One in six men with prostate cancer experience depression (Fervaha et al. 2019)

"Have you tried to talk to him about this?" Lisa asked gently.

Pauline shook her head. She was scared about what his response might be.

"Can I ask why you haven't talked to him?

Pauline sat silent for a few minutes and then looked up at Lisa. "It feels to me like it did when I tried to talk to my first husband. He also cut me out, didn't talk to me, and this time I didn't want to stir the pot, if you know what I mean. His behavior was similar to my ex who started to stay at work later and later . . . at least I thought he was staying at work."

"And what was he doing?"

"He was having an affair!" Pauline's voice was loud, and she covered her mouth with her hand. "Sorry. I didn't mean to shout. But how could I not see the signs?" She was sobbing now, and Lisa waited until her sobs turned to sniffs.

"But this is not the same relationship. It sounds to me like your husband may be depressed. You said that you haven't asked him that, but you need to. I know it's scary, but how you're feeling now is scary too. And asking may be the only way he gets help."

Pauline nodded. Lisa was right, she was scared, but she needed to address the situation with Al.

No one ever said it was easy to talk about sensitive topics! There are suggestions and tips in chapter 1 that may be helpful when your partner is reluctant to talk.

Lisa and Pauline talked for a few minutes more. When she talked to the nurse practitioner, she felt brave enough to talk to Al, but as she drove home, she felt her courage disappear. When she got home, she found Al sitting on the couch in the living room. He was staring out the window, his posture that of an old man. Pauline stood at the entrance to the living room for a few minutes, trying to calm her nerves.

"Honey, Al, can I ask you something?" Al didn't turn to look at her. Had he heard or was he ignoring her? She cleared her throat and re-peated herself. Once again there was no response from her husband. She forced herself to walk toward him; she wanted to touch his shoulder, but she remembered how he had jumped away from her earlier that day. She stood in front of him and asked him the same question again, "Al, can I ask you something?"

He looked up at her, his eyes narrow and a pained look on his face.

"Is there something wrong? Are you in pain? Has something hap-pened?" Her voice was shrill, and she could hear the desperation in her words.

"Why should there be anything wrong? Can't a man have some peace in his own home? I left work early to get some rest at home and yet, here you are . . ." He didn't finish the sentence and started to get up off the couch.

This time Pauline was not going to be ignored and she put out her hand to stop him from moving. "I think you're depressed and . . ."

This time it was she who did not finish the sentence. Al's response to her was loud and hurtful. Within minutes they were having a fight unlike any other in the ten years of their marriage. They used words that they had never used before. Their voices were loud and harsh but neither cared. The fight lasted for more than twenty minutes. Each time one of them tried to move to another room, the other followed, their anger greater with the attempt at distance. Neither raised their hands toward the other, but their words hurt more than a push or slap ever could.

Just as quickly as the fight started, it was over. One minute they were screaming at each other, their faces contorted with rage, tears running down their face, and the next they were both exhausted and shocked at the violence of their language and their anger at each other.

Arguments, themselves, are not a significant risk to a relationship. Most couples argue at some point. But *how* they argue is key to maintaining a healthy relationship. Read about negative responses in chapter 1.

In the aftermath of the fight, things were awkward. They were polite to each other, in the way that strangers sharing living space would be. They said "please" and "thank you" for small actions, but they both kept their feelings to themselves. On the next Friday evening, Pauline came home and went straight to the fridge to take out a bottle of wine. Since Al's diagnosis they had reduced their alcohol use significantly and the same bottle of wine had been in the fridge for months. She stood at the kitchen counter, wineglass in hand, the cold liquid frosting the glass. She still had her coat on, and her purse remained slung over her shoulder.

"That bad, huh?" remarked Al, referring to her day at work. It was the first time that he had said something that suggested that he noticed something about her.

Pauline hesitated for just a second before replying. "Quite the week."

"I guess we should talk about . . . well, everything?" Al sounded contrite, and his voice was soft.

"Yes, we should. Let me change into something comfortable first."

When she returned to the kitchen, she found Al sitting at the kitchen counter, a glass of wine in front of him. She was nervous, but his statement suggested an opening for them to really talk about the fight and hopefully everything else. Neither of them seemed ready to start talking; they sipped their wine, not looking at each other. When Pauline glanced at her husband, he was looking at her, and they both laughed.

"Okay, I'll go first," said Al. He took a big gulp of his wine and started coughing. When she reached out to pat his back, he motioned for her that he was fine. This small action hurt her feelings and she fought to keep silent. "Paul . . . you asked me if I was depressed. No, you actually *told* me that I was depressed and well, I reacted to that."

"I'll say!" Pauline couldn't help herself from reacting, "Sorry . . . please carry on."

"So that pushed a button for me. I haven't been feeling great and well, you sounded like I had done something wrong, and that's why I lashed out."

"That's not what I meant!" Pauline's voice was louder than she intended, "I've been really worried about you. You were just gone! You were here but you were gone!"

Al felt his anger coming back. He tried to keep his voice under control but within seconds they were fighting again. This time Al left the house, the kitchen door banging against the wall. It had happened again, thought Pauline, why could they not have a decent discussion about things anymore? She finished the bottle of wine and went to bed. She didn't hear her husband come home, but the next morning when she woke up, her head aching, she saw that he had slept on the couch. That had never happened before, and the sight of the rumpled blanket on the living room floor frightened her.

When she had found out about her ex-husband's affair, there had been no discussion, no accusations, no apologies. On the day that she found the receipt from a hotel on his desk, she told him to get out, and he left. She had never seen him again, but one of her friends had told her that he had married the woman he had the affair with. He never had any interest in their daughter and, as far as she was concerned, he was part of the past; that is, until now that Al was acting just like her ex. He was angry and defensive and distant.

She had always thought that her relationship with Al was different. But these fights had her worried that something in their marriage had changed, and she was scared that there was no going back to what it was before. She had promised herself after her divorce that she would not settle for a bad relationship ever again, and Al had never given her cause to distrust him. But his distancing from her and his reluctance to talk about his feelings made her not trust herself, and this was not a good feeling.

They got through the rest of the weekend, in silence and avoiding each other. On Monday morning she called Lisa, her nurse practitioner, and asked for a referral to a marriage counselor. She didn't feel comfortable seeing the psychologist at the college health service and wanted to see someone in the community. Lisa gave her the contact information for a Dr. Albert, a psychologist and marriage therapist, whose practice was in a bedroom community about thirty minutes away. She called immediately and left a message for Dr. Albert to call her back.

She waited all day for a call back but heard nothing. She checked her phone compulsively and was about to give up when, on her drive home, Dr. Albert called her. The psychologist sounded young, and Pauline was worried that she would not be a good match for what was troubling her. But Dr. Albert said that she had an opening later that week, and Pauline agreed to the appointment. She thought about telling Al that she was going to see someone for help but decided that she would wait and see how the appointment went.

The next two days were a repeat of the days following the huge fight with Al. He slept in their bed again but was watching TV when Pauline fell asleep. He was still sleeping, or at least pretending to be, when she got up in the morning. The bookstore opened later in the morning, and they had always had coffee together before she left for work, but not now. Any residual anger that Pauline might have felt after their two fights had dissolved, but she now just felt an overwhelming sadness.

The hours went by until the afternoon of her appointment with the psychologist. She left work in plenty of time and found herself in the parking lot of the building where Dr. Albert had her office. She sat in the car, watching the minutes pass on the clock, until it was five minutes before the hour. Dr. Albert's office was on the ground floor and there was a note on the office door, instructing people to wait until they were called into the office. There were two chairs next to the door, but Pauline was too nervous to sit down. At exactly one minute before her appointment time, the office door opened and a woman about the same age as her, introduced herself as Dr. Albert. Pauline felt herself relax just a tiny bit; she was relieved that Dr. Albert was not as young as her voice suggested.

The appointment went well; Dr. Albert was a good listener and she encouraged Pauline to verbalize her feelings. When Pauline finally stopped talking, her face flushed and her breathing fast, Dr. Albert asked her what she wanted to do about the situation. Pauline didn't know how to answer—surely the psychologist should be the one to make suggestions about resolving the issues in her relationship?

"Well, I guess that we, my husband and I, need help to get through this."

"Do you think he would be willing to do some counseling with you?" Dr. Albert responded.

Pauline, sighed. She was not sure he would be willing to talk about his feelings to a stranger; after all, he wasn't willing to talk to her! She shook her head.

"Why don't you write him a letter, Pauline?" the psychologist asked gently. "From what you've described, recent conversations have turned into an argument. Often writing down how you feel is clearer than talking about your feelings, and for the person reading the letter, an immediate and potentially reactive response is not what usually happens."

Pauline thought about this for a moment. In the early days of their relationship, she used to send him cards and letters; she remembered how romantic things were back then and it made her feel even sadder. He had not responded with words of his own but had given her books of poetry with pages that reflected his feelings marked by sticky notes. She told Dr. Albert this, blushing as she recounted the early days of their relationship.

Dr. Albert smiled as she listened. "Yes, we all long for those days of romance and giant gestures."

And with that, the appointment was over. Pauline drove home, her head full of the words that she thought she could put down on paper. Before she changed her mind, she sat down at the kitchen counter and started to write. Her hand started to ache, and she stretched; thirty minutes had passed, and she still had her coat on! She folded the pages and left them on the counter where Al would find them when he got home.

Writing a letter, by hand rather than texting or emailing, is an effective way to express feelings in a thoughtful way. The process of writing may be cathartic and help you process your feelings, and receiving the letter will help your partner to process their response.

She waited for Al to return from work; she was nervous and found herself pacing through the house. When she heard the kitchen door open, she walked quickly to their bedroom where she waited for him to come upstairs. She tried to focus on his movement downstairs, but the house was silent. She hoped he was reading the letter and when she heard his footsteps on the stairs, she felt her heart beating faster. His footsteps hesitated at the top of the stairs and she held her breath as he approached their bedroom. Then he was standing there, the pages of the letter she had written in his hand. She couldn't read the expression on his face, and for an instant she wanted to flee.

"Paul . . . my love . . ." His first words filled her with relief and her eyes with tears. He wasn't angry! "I had no idea," he continued. "Divorce is the last thing on my mind! I am so sorry that the thought even entered your mind! I love you. I love what we have! And I am so, so sorry that we have landed up here. What can do to fix this? I don't want you to feel like you're alone. I'm so sorry."

When she stopped crying, and with his arms around her, Pauline told him that she had been to get help and that she thought that maybe he should go and see Dr. Albert to talk about how he was feeling. She felt his arms stiffen and he started to shift his body away from her. She held onto him tighter; it had taken courage to write the letter and she was determined that he—they—needed help. She looked at his face, her expression pleading with him to agree.

And he did.

One week later he went to see Dr. Albert. Pauline had told him that the psychologist was about their age and a good listener. She didn't admit that the letter had been Dr. Albert's suggestion. Some things needed to be kept secret!

He came home after the appointment and didn't say much about it other than to ask Pauline if she would be willing to go back to see Dr. Albert, this time with him.

"Of course!" was her reply; she felt hopeful for the first time in ages.

She was not sure what to expect at the next appointment. Dr. Albert asked them to face each other on the couch and Pauline was surprised when Al reached over and took her hand. He had not said anything to her in the car about what he was feeling, but maybe he was just as nervous as she was! The psychologist thanked them both for their willingness to work on their relationship and asked Al if he was ready to talk to his wife.

Al cleared his throat. "Paul, when I came to see Dr. Albert by myself, she asked me about my family, you know, my parents and stuff. But you're my family now, I want you to know that . . ."

Pauline nodded.

"Well, I never told you much about my parents, and there's a reason for that. You know that my father was in the military, right? And that he fought in Korea? What I didn't tell you is that he didn't die when I was a kid."

Pauline was holding her breath as he talked. She knew very little about his childhood but she had always thought that what she knew was accurate. Al hardly talked about his childhood and frankly, she hadn't really asked him much about it.

"The truth is that one day he went to work and he never came back. One day he was there and the next he was gone, and we never found out what happened to him. We never talked about it again. There were whispers in the small town where we lived but we ignored them as best we could. My mother was overwhelmed with the three of us. She had to find a job and we just had to manage. We didn't have much and we often went to bed hungry. One night she heard me crying in bed. It was winter and there was no heat in the house, and I was cold and hungry and she . . . well, she gave me the beating of my life. She was crying but she didn't stop until my big brother woke up and pulled her off me. I never cried again, not in her house."

His face was expressionless. Pauline squeezed his hand, but he did not react.

Dr. Albert looked at Pauline, who had tears streaming down her cheeks, but Al seemed to not notice.

"Does that help you to understand your husband a little more?"

Pauline nodded. What he had described explained a lot, not only about their current dynamics but also about their relationship, in general. He had never really been open about sharing his feelings. Somewhere deep inside was that little boy, scared and beaten for showing weakness.

"That helps . . . thank you, honey. But why did you not tell me that before? And is this the only reason that you've been, well, different now? You've recovered so well, and your doctor said that everything was good. I don't understand."

Dr. Albert waited to see if Al would respond, but he was staring out the window.

Pauline spoke before the psychologist could say any more. "Al? Is there something else going on? You've lost weight, you're sleeping more, you seem uninterested in everything. You're a different person these days! You are not the same person that I fell in love with and I'm lonely and I'm scared!"

Her husband didn't answer.

Dr. Albert got straight to the point. "Al, do you think you're depressed?"

This provoked a response in Al who seemed startled by the question. "Depressed? I . . . I don't know. Why would I be depressed?"

Most men are socialized to not show weakness or emotions, and this means that they often find it difficult to both express their feelings and/or ask for help. Some men will express anger and behave in an aggressive manner instead of admitting, to themselves and others, that they are scared or depressed. (Rice et al. 2018)

Dr. Albert asked Al questions about his sleep, appetite, and activities. He admitted that he had not been sleeping well and was not interested in food or anything else, for that matter. He blushed as he answered "yes" to the question about sex: he had lost all interest and was afraid that Pauline had noticed.

"Of course, I noticed!" Pauline could not help herself from responding. Pauline tried to keep calm, but it was useless. All her insecurities from her first marriage were centered on sex, or the lack of it, and if Al thought she would not notice, well he didn't understand her at all. "I thought you were having an affair! You ignored me and we didn't talk! All we did was fight! You stayed at work later and later and you stopped sleeping in our bed but most of all, you were distant, gone, somewhere else! How do you think I would NOT notice?"

Pauline was crying now, openly and in that ugly cry that she hated.

Dr. Albert stepped in to control the emotions that were now out in the open. "Pauline, Al . . . let's stop for a minute and everyone take a deep breath. It really does sound to me like you're depressed, Al. There is nothing to be ashamed of, and this can be treated in various ways. Would you like to hear about what you can do to manage this?"

Pauline felt vindicated but also angry. She had asked Al if he was depressed, and he had responded with anger. The hurtful words from the fight they had after she asked came flooding back and she fought to control them.

"Okay, Dr. Albert, what do I need to do?" Al's voice was barely audible as he looked at the psychologist.

Treatments for depression include medications (anti-depressants) and/or counseling (psychotherapy). While antidepressants are effective in treating depression, many cause sexual side effects that may compound the sexual dysfunction associated with prostate cancer treatment. (Fervaha et al. 2019)

Al listened, his eyes fixed on the psychologist's face. He felt some relief that it was all out in the open. He was depressed and he felt guilty that he had pushed Pauline away when she had tried to help. He didn't know why he had done that, and he hated to see her so frustrated and sad and angry with him. He needed to apologize to her for his actions and his words, but first he needed to think about what he was going to do to feel better.

Pauline felt better too, but she also recognized that there was more work to be done. Secrets and avoidance had led to misunderstandings and arguments. They needed to learn to be more open with each other; and, as much as she loved him and he loved her, they had a lot to learn about communication.

CONCLUSION

Communication lies at the center of relationships; talking about sensitive topics can be challenging for even the happiest couples. Most couples make assumptions about what each other is thinking; this is a natural extension of knowing each other well. But we also get it wrong! The suggestions in this chapter are not all there is to improve communication with your partner, and finding professional help may be the most useful step when you find that your relationship is challenged.

Reflective Questions

After reading this chapter:

- What would you do if you found that your partner/spouse is withdrawing and you are not sure what is happening?
- What strategies do you and your partner/spouse use to ensure open communication?
- What have you learned from the suggestions in this chapter about improving communication with your partner/spouse?
- If you were to write a letter to your partner/spouse about any changes in your relationship after his diagnosis of prostate cancer, what would you write?

REFERENCES

Fervaha, G., J. P. Izard, D. A. Tripp, S. Rajan, D. P. Leong, and D. R. Siemens. 2019. "Depression and prostate cancer: A focused review for the clinician." *Urologic Oncology* 37 (4): 282–88. doi: 10.1016/j.urolonc.2018.12.020.

Rice, S. M., J. L. Oliffe, M. T. Kelly, P. Cormie, S. Chambers, J. S. Ogrodniczuk, and D. Kealy. 2018. "Depression and prostate cancer: Examining comorbidity and male-specific symptoms." *American Journal of Men's Health* 12 (6): 1864–72. doi: 10.1177/1557988318784395.

Sefik, E., B. Gunlusoy, A. Eker, S. Celik, Y. Ceylan, A. Koskderelioglu, I. Basmaci, and T. Degirmenci. 2020. "Anxiety and depression associated with a positive prostate biopsy result: A comparative, prospective cohort study." *International Brazilian Journal of Urology* 46 (6): 993–1005. doi: 10.1590/s1677-5538.ibju.2019.0719.

Chapter Eleven

The Role of Support Groups

*"It's Easier to Talk to
Someone Who's Been Through This"*

Support groups for men with prostate cancer are common; some include partners who participate in part of the meeting, while others have separate meetings for partners. These groups have been shown to be helpful for both the men and their partners. In this chapter, the reader will learn how the spouse of a man with prostate cancer finds support from an online forum for women whose partner/spouse has prostate cancer.

Cheryl, age sixty, has been married to Donald, who is four years older, for almost forty years. Donald is the editor of the local newspaper in their small town, about an hour outside Seattle. Cheryl had to close her yarn store soon after the start of the COVID-19 pandemic, but she was able to switch to home deliveries and for this she was grateful. Sales of yarn and knitting patterns were good, initially, when almost all her regular customers were forced to stay home. But business had dropped off and she is not sure how much longer she could hang on. She had to let go her longtime assistant, who she misses, but it was not financially viable to keep her on. She feels guilty about this and worries constantly about the future of the store and the financial implications of closing her business.

They have no children, and travel has always been a mutual love; they had plans to travel to each continent on the planet when they were both retired. Now those plans are in jeopardy; closing her store will cost her money and dry up her source of income. Because of the many travel restrictions since the start of the pandemic, Donald decided that he would delay his retirement; there didn't seem to be much point in retiring only to sit at home.

Donald had surgery for low-risk prostate cancer in May 2020. He was originally supposed to have the surgery in early April, but it was delayed due to the pandemic. The surgery went well; he was discharged after just two days and was happy for that, as he was worried about getting infected with COVID-19 while in the hospital. He recovered well, and once the catheter came out, he was almost back to his normal self. He had been working from home before the surgery and, within three weeks, he was back at his desk in his home office, busy with the day-to-day activities that kept the newspaper running. The only wrinkle was that he still had a lot of leakage. He was thankful that he didn't have to go to the office because he needed to be close to the bathroom. Cheryl was at a loss as to what to do about what was obviously bothering her husband. She tried asking him if she could help in any way, and he barked at her.

"I'm fine! I'm not a baby! Stop asking me how I am!"

Cheryl was shocked at his response. They had always shared everything with each other; not having children had made them close, as they only had each other to lean on. They lived far from their siblings and were used to sharing holidays with their small circle of friends or even just each other. She had gone with him to the appointment when he learned that he had prostate cancer, but that was the last time that she accompanied him to any appointments. She understood that because of COVID-19, there were limits to the number of "companions" (strange word for a person's partner!) that could accompany someone to medical appointments. She was not allowed to visit him in the hospital after his surgery, and this caused her a lot of stress. He had his phone with him, but he slept most of the time; when he didn't answer her calls, she panicked and called the nurses' station. When he was discharged, she was relieved, but that didn't last long. There was obviously something wrong, but he wasn't talking to her about it.

The next day, she talked to her former assistant, Sara, on the phone. Over the years they had become good friends, and this was one of the reasons that she felt so guilty when she had to let her go. Sara insisted that she understood the reason why she was no longer employed but Cheryl continued to feel bad. They talked to each other regularly and Cheryl tried to steer their conversation away from anything related to the shop. This call was no different, and when they ran out of conversation, Cheryl found herself describing what was going on at home.

"I don't know what to do!" Cheryl's voice was wobbly. "You know how close we are . . . how close we *were*. He won't tell me what's going on, and I feel so helpless."

"That must be horrible, Cheryl. You two are the last couple I would expect anything like this to happen to!"

"That's what I always thought!" Cheryl was crying now and she couldn't say anything more.

"Have you talked to anyone else about what is happening?"

Cheryl sniffed and shook her head, then realized that Sara couldn't see her. "No, you are the first person and really the only one I trust. If Donald knew that I had talked to you . . ." As she said the words, she realized that she had betrayed Donald's confidence and he would be furious with her. She instantly regretted telling Sara but part of her, a very small part, felt lighter now that she had told someone. "Please, please, don't tell anyone what I told you!" Cheryl pleaded with her friend. "Donald would be just devastated if he thought that anyone knew."

"I would never tell anyone! Trust me, I know how horrible this is for you. Remember when I had that health scare? I told you and I knew you wouldn't tell anyone. In hindsight I don't know why I wanted to keep it a secret, but I told you, and you were such a great help."

Cheryl did remember. Sara had never married and she had no family other than some cousins that she was not close to. When she needed to have a biopsy after they saw something on a routine mammogram, Sara fell to pieces. Cheryl was scared for her assistant and had supported her in any way she could. That was when their relationship changed to one of friendship and they had become confidants. In her heart, she trusted her and knew that Sara wouldn't say anything to anyone about what she had told her.

Cheryl ended the call when she heard Donald leaving his home office and walking toward the kitchen where she was sitting. He looked unhappy, and she almost asked him if she could help him, but she thought better of it. She was not in the mood for an argument or harsh words. They had barely talked since his outburst the day before, and so she kept her voice light as she asked him what he felt like for dinner.

"Make whatever you want," was his response, "I'm not really hungry."

He was searching for something in the fridge as he said this, and Cheryl stared at him. If he wasn't hungry, why was he looking for something to eat? Once again, she kept quiet. This was the worst part of what was happening to him; it was affecting their relationship and she hated this feeling of walking on eggshells around him. But what was she supposed to do?

There are times when silence makes the loudest noise.
Not sharing a problem with one's partner can become
part of a much larger issue with loss of emotional connection and distancing.

Donald found what he was looking for, a plastic container of nuts that she had forgotten about, then went back to his office without saying a word. Cheryl sat at the kitchen table, staring out of the window. She knew that she needed to do something, but what? She had been scrolling through her Facebook page before the call with Sara, and as she went back to the website, a thought occurred to her. What if she searched for information about prostate cancer and its effects on men? She wanted to hit herself over the head—why had she not thought of this before? She had been so preoccupied with her store and keeping her business going that she had not bothered to learn anything about what Donald might go through! She quickly typed her question and immediately the screen filled with links to websites.

She clicked on the first one on the screen. As she started to read, she realized how much she didn't know about his cancer. At the one appointment she went to with her husband it sounded like he had to have surgery; there was no discussion about anything else. Donald had accepted the recommendation from the doctor and had signed consent for surgery immediately. Then there was the delay because of COVID-19, her panic about closing her store to customers and getting the word out about home delivery, and, finally, he had the operation. When she read about the side effects of the surgery, she felt her heart sink. That was what was happening to Donald! He was having problems with his bladder, and she had ignored this! She went back to the list of websites and found one that talked about the effects of cancer treatment on the couple and there it was, the words almost jumping off the screen—prostate cancer is a couples' disease with implications for the relationship!

Prostate cancer is often referred to as a "couples' disease," in part because, as a disease affecting men, those who are partnered find themselves relying heavily on their partner/spouse for support.

Cheryl sat, staring at the screen, her thoughts jumbled. No, they had not had sex since the surgery, but she thought that was because he was still recovering. She had not considered that he might be having problems with erections or the other side effects that she had just now read about. And the realization that he was having problems with his bladder made her feel guilty that she had not been more supportive or had offered him help. But how was she supposed to help if he didn't open up to her? She resolved to try talking to him, maybe after dinner, but she wanted to keep reading.

Another website that she found included a section on how the partner of the man with prostate cancer needed support too. This was the first website she had found that had a focus on the partner, and she felt tears come to her eyes. She kept reading—about the need for communication between the couple and the importance of self-care for the partner—and she felt an overwhelming sense of relief mixed with sadness. But she also realized that she had let her husband down by not educating herself about his cancer and treatment.

Something else she read on one of the websites made her think about what Donald was going through and his need for support and education. The website had links to organizations that had support groups for men with prostate cancer. Did Donald know about these? There was so much she wanted to talk to him about, but she was nervous about how he would respond.

Support groups for men with prostate cancer have a long history and have been shown to be useful as they allow men to share experiences and to offer advice and support to each other. (De Silva et al. 2018)

That weekend, the perfect opportunity to talk arrived in the form of an invitation to visit friends who lived two hours away. Grace and Dennis were the kind of friends that every couple needed. The two couples had been friends for ten years, having met on a Caribbean cruise. They had a lot in common; a love of good wine and travel, similar political views, no children, and a mutual dislike of food critics. They had shared vacations over the years, and even though they had not seen each other over the months of the COVID-19 pandemic, regular phone calls and the occasional virtual wine tasting on Zoom had kept their friendship close. Donald and Cheryl were not worried about the risk of COVID-19 when visiting the other couple. They were all working from home and had limited outside activities for months. They agreed that they would each have a COVID-19 test before the weekend, and they had all tested negative.

Cheryl was excited about the weekend; she was looking forward to good conversation but also to having uninterrupted time to talk to her husband on the drive. What she had read on the websites she visited had given her a lot of ideas about how she and Donald could communicate and what she had learned about the side effects of his treatment had softened her irritation with him. She just hoped that he would not get angry with her; after all, he was going to be driving and she didn't want him to get distracted. But she had a plan for how she was going to introduce the topic of a support group to him. She believed that if he would agree to attend one of these groups, he would be better able to cope with whatever was bothering him.

She had packed a thermos of hot chocolate for the ride and, at the last minute, added a container of frozen shortbread to the bag containing four bottles of wine for the dinner that she and Grace had planned. The men had taken care of the wine list for the dinner, and Donald's contribution was from deep in their wine collection under the stairs. They had each packed a small bag with their clothes and toiletries and were ready to leave thirty minutes before their planned departure time. For the first time in months, Donald looked relaxed and even happy. Cheryl had second thoughts about trying to talk to him about what was bothering him. Why ruin the weekend before it really began, she thought to herself, maybe the conversation could wait until they drove home on Monday?

Couples often deal with problems by keeping silent and pretending to ignore what is happening. But not talking about things that are bothering you only makes the problem grow. Eventually the silence will be broken, not infrequently by an argument.

From the moment they arrived at their friends' home, it was like they had seen each other only one month ago. They fell into easy conversation, the women in the kitchen and the men in the den. Cheryl brought out the shortbread they had not eaten in the car, and Grace made coffee. The men joined them in the kitchen and they continued to talk, sharing tales about how they had all navigated the pandemic.

"We're going for a walk, ladies" Dennis announced as they finished their coffee, the shortbread crumbs scattered over the kitchen table. "Do you want to join us?"

Cheryl and Grace looked at each other and simultaneously shook their heads.

"Okay then, see you later . . . maybe lunchtime?"

With that the two men left the house, the front door banging closed behind them. The women sat in silence for a few minutes, their thoughts hidden from the other.

Grace looked at her friend, the expression on her face serious. "Cheryl? What are you thinking? You look so worried."

Cheryl couldn't answer. She felt the tears beginning to fill her eyes and her throat felt like she had swallowed a rock. Grace looked surprised; her friend was on the verge of tears. What was going on?

"It's nothing . . . don't worry about me. I'm fine." Cheryl shook her head as if to physically get rid of whatever was bothering her. Grace decided not to push the issue and the women got up and began preparing lunch for when the men returned. Grace and Dennis had a beautiful home and the dining room table was decorated as if they were having a fancy dinner party. There were flowers that matched the color scheme of the table settings, and an air of luxury permeated the room. When the men returned, they washed their hands and sat down quickly at the table.

"What's for lunch, honey?" asked Dennis, his hand on the silverware at his place.

"Do you think of anything other than food?" shouted Grace from the kitchen where she and Cheryl were plating the Waldorf salad and slicing the warm baguette.

"You know the answer to that!" laughed Dennis, noticing that his friend was not smiling as he usually would. They had not talked much on the walk, other than the occasional comment about the weather or the state of the forest. That too was unusual; Donald was normally eager to talk politics or international affairs.

Grace was an excellent cook, and she had baked brownies for dessert that she served warm with vanilla ice cream.

"I need a nap after that" joked Dennis, patting his stomach.

"I think we all do," replied Cheryl. She was feeling the strain of putting on a happy face for her friends.

Donald looked like he could also use a break and he excused himself from the table, saying that he needed to check up on something related to the newspaper. The atmosphere was awkward now; it was obvious that something was different about Cheryl and Donald. Cheryl got up and started to clear the table but Grace waved her off.

"You've had a long day with the drive and all. Go and have a lie-down, and we can have tea later this afternoon."

When they were alone, Grace looked at her husband with a confused look on her face and he shrugged his shoulders. "What do you think has happened? They're really tense and so different with each other." There was concern in Grace's voice. One of the things she had always admired about their friends was the way they were physically affectionate with each other. They held hands and sat close together and it was obvious to her that they were very much in love. She and Dennis did not have that kind of relationship and she was jealous that he was not demonstrative like Donald.

"Who knows, honey? Maybe they had a fight on the way here." Dennis did not seem to have noticed the distance between their friends. "But Donald was kinda quiet on our walk. But I am not going to interfere and neither should you!"

Later that afternoon, Cheryl came down to the main floor but Donald was not with her. "There's some sort of crisis at the newspaper." Cheryl volunteered, "I'm so sorry, we're awful guests."

Grace and Dennis reassured her that they understood, but they were puzzled by their friends' behavior. Things were certainly not normal.

Dennis took Donald's absence as a reason to excuse himself and went to watch golf on the TV in the den. Cheryl and Grace sat quietly at the table; Cheryl seemed far away, her gaze on her hands and her shoulders slumped. Grace took a deep breath and once again asked her friend what was wrong. She knew this was a risk; when she had asked earlier it seemed to upset her. But this time Cheryl opened up and all her worries spilled out.

"It's Donald . . . you know he had prostate cancer that was treated a couple of months ago?"

Grace nodded; Donald had called Dennis when he was diagnosed, urging his friend to get regular PSA tests. Dennis had reassured Donald that he was fine and was "good."

"He seemed to be okay after the surgery. He was only in the hospital for two days and he seemed to be doing really well."

Grace nodded; the men had kept in contact as Donald recovered and she thought that everything was fine now.

Cheryl hesitated; she was scared to talk about her husband but she was desperate to talk to someone. "I don't know what's going on with him but he's different now, and he won't tell me what's bothering him."

Grace reached over and put her hand on Cheryl's. "Cheryl, I don't know if I ever told you this, but remember that cruise when we first met? Well, that was to celebrate my first year after cancer treatment."

Cheryl was shocked; Grace had never said anything about having had cancer.

"Yeah, I had breast cancer. It was tough, that year. And Dennis wanted us to do something to mark the milestone of a year after treatment. I was not sure that there was anything to celebrate, but you know my husband. He's very persuasive!"

"I had no idea." Cheryl did not know what to say. She wanted to ask so many questions, but she didn't want to seem nosy.

"I was lucky, I guess" Grace continued, "I had surgery to remove the cancer and then radiation. I didn't need to have chemo, so I didn't lose my hair but it was still a tough year, going through all that . . ." The memory of her distant cancer, more than a decade before, cast a shadow over her face. But she was not finished. "Dennis took it hard. He was great of course, he supported me in so many ways. But I could see that he was struggling. He had no one to lean on, and that was difficult. That's one of the downsides of not having kids, I guess. It was just us and he was shielding me from his worries."

Cheryl nodded. This was exactly how she was feeling!

The partner of the man with prostate cancer often has unmet needs for information about the disease, treatment, and how to support him. Partners need information and validation of what they are experiencing. (Evertsen and Wolkenstein 2010)

"One of the things that really helped him was a support group for the partners of women with breast cancer that was offered by the cancer center where I had my radiation. Have you thought of that for you?"

Now that they were talking it was as if a floodgate had been opened. Cheryl told her friend how lonely she felt and how ill-prepared she was to support Donald. Grace listened, her hand still on her friend's hand.

"Have you looked at support groups for spouses where you live?" Grace asked softly.

Cheryl shook her head. She hadn't told Grace how difficult it had been to keep her business afloat during the pandemic or how hard it had been to let Sara go. She hadn't had the energy to do anything other than focusing on the store and now she felt guilty that she hadn't paid attention to what Donald was going through.

"I feel awful." Cheryl had tears pouring down her face.

Grace tried to comfort her friend. "Remember what they tell you when you fly? Put on your oxygen mask before helping someone else."

Cheryl smiled through her tears. "Oh, I barely remember going on a plane."

"Me either!" Grace responded, "Would you consider going to a support group?"

Cheryl sat for a moment, thinking about the question. "I don't know . . . Donald has not gone to one. I don't know how he would feel."

It is not unusual for the partner of the man to be sensitive to his feelings and this impacts their willingness to seek support for themselves. Some men may experience stigma as a result of their cancer, particularly if they have incontinence or sexual problems, because of how these side effects relate to common conceptions of masculinity, (Wood et al. 2019)

"I went to a support group after I was diagnosed," Grace told her friend. "It felt weird to go and bare my soul, or at least that is what I thought happened at these groups. But it was nothing like that. I met some amazing women and they helped me deal with the emotions that I was experiencing. The meetings were part information from professionals and a big part was sharing what we were going through. They really helped."

"Donald has never talked about anything like this being offered. And because of COVID-19, I couldn't go with him to his appointments. I wonder if he even knows about these support groups? They sound like a good idea."

"Dennis went to one for partners of women with breast cancer. I had to twist his arm and the nurse navigator who had helped me when I was diagnosed was quite insistent that he needed to go. She had told him in the beginning that men often hide their feelings and the support group was a place where he could admit to those feelings. He was so angry after I was diagnosed, and I felt like his anger was directed at *me*! The support of the other men really helped him."

Grace and Cheryl continued to talk into the early evening. It felt good to be able to share her concerns, and Cheryl realized that she had ignored her own feelings about Donald's cancer. This had affected her too, but she was so focused on her business that she had pushed down her worries and even neglected her husband. The guilt she felt was overwhelming. But along with the guilt was the realization that she and Donald needed to talk. She had not said anything on the way to their friends because she didn't want to ruin the weekend, but she had to talk to him on the way home.

On the drive home after the weekend with their friends, she started the conversation. She was nervous but resolved; their relationship depended on it. Donald was more relaxed than he had been in while, he had the radio tuned to a soft rock station and was moving his head in time to the music. Cheryl hated to ruin his mood, but she took a deep breath and started to talk.

Donald refused to engage in any discussion. His jaw was clenched and the muscles on the side of his face twitched. He was staring at the road ahead and the skin over his knuckles was white with tension.

"This has nothing to do with you!" he muttered.

Cheryl was shocked at first, but grew angry within minutes. She fought to control her response to him, but it was no use; she was furious and her anger erupted.

"How dare you? How can you ignore *my* feelings? This is not just about you! This has everything to do with me, with us! Do you honestly think that I can't see that something is bothering you? I have been agonizing about how I can help you for weeks and all you can say is that this has nothing to do with me!"

Cheryl was so angry that she was crying, big sobs that made her feel like she was choking. But her husband did not say anything or slow down or pull off the road. He kept driving, and Cheryl turned her face to the window, the scenery flashing by in a blur of green trees and fields. They got home in what seemed like record time, and probably was, as Donald was driving way above the speed limit. Donald stormed off to his home office, leaving Cheryl to bring in their bags. She dumped the bags just inside the door and went directly to her laptop. Within minutes, she found the number of a social worker at the hospital where Donald had his surgery. It was late so she left a message for the social worker to call her back in the morning.

Cheryl did not sleep well that night. She was still angry with her husband, who slept on the couch in the den. They barely looked at each other in the morning, and when Cheryl's phone rang, she stepped outside on the deck to answer the call. It was the social worker and they had a brief conversation. She anticipated what the social worker would say: due to the COVID-19 pandemic, in-person support groups were not possible. Cheryl was disappointed and was about to end the call when they social worker told her that there were online support groups that he could participate in, and there were also some for partners.

"I'll email you a list of support groups for partners and family members that are available online. Many people actually prefer these—you don't have to leave the house to participate, and you'll meet people from all over!"

Cheryl was not sure about this; she thanked the social worker and logged on to her email. Within minutes, there was a *bing*, and there was the email with a long list of websites. Cheryl was about to delete the email, but as the cursor hovered over the delete icon, she thought better of it. She was not ready to explore this any further, but something told her that the timing might be better later.

Health care providers see the benefits of participation in prostate cancer support groups (Garrett et al. 2014). Men with prostate cancer describe how the support that they receive counteracts the loneliness that they experience (Dunn et al. 2018). Online support groups also provide support for spouses and family members (Ihrig et al. 2019).

The rest of the day crawled by; business was slow, and Chery wondered if she should be opening the store now that COVID-19 cases were on the decline. Some other businesses had opened, but she was still worried about the spread of COVID-19 and having to police customers who weren't wearing their masks. Donald spent most of the day in his home office and she overheard him talking to the publisher of the paper about going back to in-person work. She hoped he would talk to her about that, but he did not say a word as they ate dinner, once again, in complete silence.

As she got up from the table, the food on her plate barely touched, Donald cleared his throat.

"Cheryl, hang on a moment. I have something to say."

She turned to look at him and she felt herself startle when she saw his face. He looked like he had aged ten years and as he spoke, she heard the emotion in his voice.

"I owe you a huge apology," he began, "I am *so* sorry for the way I have acted over the past weeks. My behavior is unforgiveable, and I hope you can forgive me."

Donald talked for the next ten minutes and Cheryl listened, her eyes never leaving his face. He described to her the shame he felt about the incontinence he was having and how guilty he felt for not telling her, at the start, how bad it was. He told her that he had called the surgeon who removed his prostate, and he said that it would take time for things to improve. And the publisher of the newspaper wanted staff to stop working from home, but Donald was afraid that if he went back to work, then everyone would know about his "pee problem." He said he had been trying to figure out what to do about this, and today the publisher told him that he needed to be one of the first to return to the office, to "set an example."

He gave a big sigh when he finally stopped talking. Cheryl went over to him and hugged him; it took him a few seconds, but then he hugged her back. They stayed like this for some time; Cheryl could feel Donald's heart beating against her chest and she hoped that he could feel hers. She was not sure what had changed and prompted him to apologize and tell her what he was feeling—she was just happy that it had happened.

She dug some shortbread cookies out of the freezer and made a pot of herbal tea as the cookies defrosted. They moved to the den and sat close together on the couch where Douglas had so recently slept. They didn't talk much as they sipped the tea and nibbled on the shortbread; they didn't need to, their physical closeness reflecting how they felt. There was time to talk in the days ahead.

As happy as she was that things seemed to have resolved with Donald, Grace's words had stuck in Chery's brain. The thought of getting support for herself went from interesting to tempting. What was the harm in looking into support for wives? She opened her laptop and found the email from the social worker with the list of support groups. She clicked on one of the links for support groups and, within a day she, was contacted by one of the peer-support coordinators. And as luck would have it, there was going to be a webinar on dealing with incontinence after surgery and it was just one week away! She told Donald about this over dinner; he didn't say much, but at least he didn't try to dissuade her. She thought about telling him that there was information about support groups for men on the website but did not want to start an argument.

The next week, she signed on to the webinar about incontinence. The expert who presented the information was a pelvic floor physiotherapist who seemed very knowledgeable. Cheryl was surprised to learn that there were things that Donald could do to help himself, and just waiting for improvement as the surgeon had suggested was not a good strategy. She was determined to talk to Donald about this, no matter what his response. And she wanted to join the Facebook group too! She requested membership to the group and soon had the invitation to the Facebook group. A whole new world opened for her and she found herself checking daily for messages and updates from other women who were part of the group.

One of the best things about the group was that it showed her she was not alone. Many of the women in the group were going through exactly what she was experiencing. She felt safe in posting on the site; she was assured that the women participating kept the posts confidential. They shared their frustrations and anger at what had happened to their partner and this helped her deal with her own emotions. And she was not alone in having a husband who wanted to deal with the side effects on his own! For the first time in ages, Cheryl felt like she could breathe. The worries about Donald seemed lighter now; as Grace had reminded her, she had put on her own oxygen mask and was ready to help Donald with his, if only he was willing.

CONCLUSION

The partner of the man with prostate cancer has their own need for support after his diagnosis, through the treatment phase, and beyond. Both members of the couple will deal with the challenges of the diagnosis and treatment in their own way, however, one person should not prevent the other from getting the support they need. While support groups for men with prostate cancer have existed for years, the same cannot be said for their partners. Online support groups for both men and their partners have made accessing support easier, especially for those who live in rural and remote locations.

Reflective Questions

After reading this chapter:

- Where do you draw support from?
- What kinds of support do you need most?
- How do you and your partner/spouse resolve conflicts?

REFERENCES

De Silva, D., W. Ranasinghe, T. Bandaragoda, A. Adikari, N. Mills, L. Iddamalgoda, D. Alahakoon, N. Lawrentschuk, R. Persad, E. Osipov, R. Gray, and D. Bolton. 2018. "Machine learning to support social media empowered patients in cancer care and cancer treatment decisions." *PLOS One* 13 (10): e0205855. doi: 10.1371/journal.pone.0205855.

Dunn, J., C. Casey, D. Sandoe, M. K. Hyde, M. C. Cheron-Sauer, A. Lowe, J. L. Oliffe, and S. K. Chambers. 2018. "Advocacy, support and survivorship in prostate cancer." *European Journal of Cancer Care* (English) 27 (2): e12644. doi: 10.1111/ecc.12644.

Evertsen, J. M., and A. S. Wolkenstein. 2010. "Female partners of patients after surgical prostate cancer treatment: Interactions with physicians and support needs." *BMC Family Practice* 11 (1):19. doi: 10.1186/1471-2296-11-19.

Garrett, B. M., J. L. Oliffe, J. L. Bottorff, M. McKenzie, C. S. Han, and J. S. Ogrodniczuk. 2014. "The value of prostate cancer support groups: a pilot study of primary physicians' perspectives." *BMC Family Practice* 15: 56. doi: 10.1186/1471-2296-15-56.

Ihrig, A., T. Renner, T. Muck, P. Maatz, A. Borkowetz, B. Keck, I. Maatouk, M. P. Wirth, and J. Huber. 2019. "Online support groups offer low-threshold backing for family and friends of patients with prostate cancer." *European Journal of Cancer Care* (English) 28 (2): e12982. doi: 10.1111/ecc.12982.

Wood, A., S. Barden, M. Terk, and J. Cesaretti. 2019. "Prostate cancer: The influence of stigma on quality of life and relationship satisfaction for survivors and their partners." *Journal of Psychosocial Oncology* 37 (3): 350–66. doi: 10.1080/07347332.2018.1489442.

Chapter Twelve

End-of-Life Care

"We Thought He'd Be Cured"

While many men treated for prostate cancer will live a long life and die of some other cause, some men will experience metastatic disease and die from their cancer. This is a profound experience for those who love the man, and the partner/spouse is often involved in end-of-life care. This chapter tells the story of a couple in their seventies for whom all treatments have failed, and the man is close to the end of his life. His spouse wants to care for him at home until the end, but she becomes overwhelmed and finally asks for help. Family members support her in this and, finally, a hospice nurse steps in to care for all of them.

Eli Garfield was diagnosed with metastatic prostate cancer five years ago at the age of seventy. The diagnosis came as a shock; he broke his elbow after he tripped over the garden hose, leading to an X-ray at the emergency department. The X-ray was followed by an emergency bone scan that showed cancer in the bones of his arm, as well as both hips. Eli, a retired insurance broker, had avoided doctor's appointments for years, despite his wife's insistence that he needed to take better care of himself. The irony was that Eli's wife, Trudy, was a retired pediatrician, but nothing she said could persuade him to visit a doctor. Eli's attitude was that she would know if something was wrong with him, but she was a pediatrician and her patients were children, not grown men.

Trudy was both annoyed and terrified at the same time when he was diagnosed. If he had only listened to her, over and over, through the years, he would not be in this position; a diagnosis of metastatic prostate cancer meant that there was no chance of cure. The staff at the emergency department were kind; they offered to call the couple's son, but Trudy refused. Their son John lived about an hour away; his wife, Erin, was due to have their first child in just over a week and this had been a difficult pregnancy, after years of infertility treatment. Trudy did not want anything to go wrong at this stage of Erin's pregnancy; they had longed for grandchildren for so many years.

Eli had an appointment with a medical oncologist where he was prescribed "hormone therapy" to prevent any further spread, and for two years, the cancer was under control. He didn't like the side effects of the injection he had every three months, but he persevered until his PSA started to rise again. Dr. Stone, the oncologist, then prescribed another medication, and then another when his PSA continued to rise. One year ago, they heard the news that they had been dreading; his cancer was now what they called "castrate-resistant" and was growing despite the lack of testosterone. He was offered chemotherapy and Trudy encouraged him to try this. He managed to have only one round and then refused to continue; the side effects were awful, and he was miserable.

Dr. Stone was matter of fact in his advice to Eli. If he had bone pain, they would offer him what Dr. Stone called "palliative radiation" and he could have whatever pain medication he needed, but that was all. Trudy knew that this is the way it would go, but it didn't make the words any easier to hear.

"You have some decisions to make now, Mr. Garfield. I can refer you to hospice now and they will support you and your family in the months to come. If you are not interested in their services, you can be admitted to hospital if things get too much."

Trudy looked at her husband as the doctor spoke. He appeared to not be listening and Trudy worried that he did not realize the seriousness of the situation. "Eli," she spoke softly, "Did you hear what Dr. Stone said? What do you want to do?"

"I want to go home, that's what I want to do!" Eli stood up suddenly, the chair rattling and almost falling behind him. He didn't say anything to Dr. Stone or his wife, but just walked out of the room, a slight limp making his departure somewhat awkward. She caught up to him quickly despite taking the time to apologize to Dr. Stone for Eli's behavior. She was angry with her husband but at the same time, heartbroken at what the doctor had told them. They drove home in silence.

While many men with localized prostate cancer will die of something else, those who are diagnosed with advanced or metastatic cancer will likely die of their cancer. Once the cancer has spread, treatment is aimed at controlling any symptoms the man experiences.

When they got home, Eli went straight to the den where he turned on the TV to a sports channel. He stayed there for hours, refusing dinner and any attempt by his wife to talk about what had happened that day. Trudy got ready for bed, but Eli was still sitting in the den, his eyes closed, but from his breathing she could tell he was not asleep.

"Eli, please come to bed. I promise you I won't nag or say anything, but you can't spend the night in that chair."

Eli grunted but he got up slowly, the expression on his face one of pain or perhaps just stiffness. Trudy forced herself to not say a word. She offered her arm to him as they started to walk toward the stairs, and he took it. Perhaps this was a sign that he was willing to accept her help, she thought as they climbed slowly up to their bedroom.

Nothing much changed over the next few months. Erin and John's firstborn, a little girl named Samantha, was now almost eighteen months old. Eli adored her and spent as much time with her as possible, watching her play with her toys or launching herself at any adult in the room for hugs and kisses. Trudy adored her as well; her love for little ones is what drew her to her career as a pediatrician and she marveled at her granddaughter's growing personality.

As the weeks went by, she noticed that Eli had less energy; he slept later each day and was ready for bed by 8 p.m. He didn't complain, but she knew that he was in pain, and it took all her self-control to stop herself from asking him if he needed help. It was obvious to her that he did, but he was proud. So she watched him like a hawk whenever he got up from his chair, just in case he stumbled. He had also lost weight and, as much as he tried to hide it with thick sweaters, his Adam's apple looked huge and his pants bagged around his thighs. He was also not eating much, and even though she tried to make him all his favorites, most of the food on his plate remained untouched.

Every week when John and Erin came to visit, they were shocked at Eli's decline. Erin seemed particularly upset; her father had died when she was in her early teens and she had become close to Eli soon after she and John started dating. Trudy had wanted to have a close relationship with her daughter-in-law, but Erin had been somewhat distant with her despite the many years of her relationship with John.

One Sunday when they visited, Erin asked to speak to Trudy privately. Trudy suggested that they sit outside while it was still warm enough. Once they were settled, Erin took a deep breath.

"Trudy, I need to know the truth . . . John does too. Eli looks awful! What is happening?"

Trudy had been waiting to have this conversation for some time. She was not sure why they had all avoided talking about this, but now it was out in the open. She too took a deep breath, and then she explained that Eli had stopped all treatment.

"But why?" Erin seemed shocked.

"His cancer is no longer responding to any of the treatments . . ."

"How do you know that? There must be something . . ."

Trudy shook her head. She could see the pain on Erin's face.

"I have a friend whose father had prostate cancer and he went to . . . I can't remember where . . . but they have this special treatment there! Why haven't you taken Eli to somewhere that specializes in prostate cancer?" Erin's voice was angry, and Trudy waited a few seconds to respond.

"Erin, I can see this is hard for you. I know that you love Eli, and this is not easy for any of us. Eli has tried everything that they have to offer. Dr. Stone is one of the top medical oncologists in the region. But nothing has worked, or at least worked for any amount of time. Please believe me."

The younger woman shook her head, causing the tears in her eyes to run down her cheeks. She stood up without looking at her mother-in-law and rushed back into the house. Trudy remained outside, the late afternoon sun casting long shadows over the grass.

It can be difficult for family members to accept that someone they love is not eligible for, or has refused, more treatment. Refusing more treatment also contradicts the idea of the person with cancer as a fighter who will do whatever is necessary to "beat" cancer.

When Trudy went back into the house, John and Erin were saying their goodbyes to Eli. Little Samantha was crying and holding out her arms to Eli for one more hug and kiss. Her husband had tears in his eyes as he reached for the toddler, his face reflecting his exhaustion after their visit. Trudy stood in the doorway of the den, her heart aching at the scene in front of her. When they finally left, the sound of Samantha's crying lessening slightly, Eli lay back in his chair and fell asleep.

Trudy busied herself tidying the kitchen. Something had shifted in Eli and she was not sure what that meant. Yes, he was more tired and, yes, he had lost more weight, but it was something else and she could not figure out what it was. When she asked him if he had any pain, he always said that he did not. She wondered if he was depressed, but he denied this too. He had never been someone who asked for help, and she thought that perhaps this was what had changed; he now needed help with so much and it was difficult for him to ask for or accept assistance.

Eli slept right through what would have been dinnertime. Trudy stood at the kitchen counter, spooning yogurt into her mouth without tasting what she was eating. She hated eating alone at the table but watching Eli push his food around the plate was painful. She did not know how to get him to eat more, and his weight loss bothered her because it somehow reflected on her ability to care for him.

She woke him gently; he seemed confused and pushed her away. She almost fell but managed to stay upright, her heart beating fast. For a few seconds, he stared at her as if he was looking at a stranger. But then he shook his head and gave her a small smile.

"Is it morning?" he asked.

"Not yet," she replied, trying to keep her voice under control. "You fell asleep in the chair and you missed dinner. I'll go and make you something light . . . maybe some toast . . . and then we can go to bed."

Eli nodded his thanks and sat in the chair looking quite content. He ate the toast slowly, crumbs falling onto his lap, and then allowed Trudy to help him up out of the chair. He held tight to her forearm as they walked toward the stairs, his gait unsteady. They managed the first three stairs, but he faltered on the next one and they almost fell. Trudy tried to brace herself against the wall and she felt a muscle in her back go into spasm. This was all she needed, she muttered to herself, and she motioned to Eli that she needed to rest for just a moment.

"I'm so sorry!" Eli almost shouted, "Did you hurt yourself? I'm use-less! I might as well be dead . . ."

"You stop that right this minute!" Trudy's voice was shrill. "Say-ing things like that is not helpful! Give me a minute and we can continue . . ."

> It is not unusual for men with advanced disease to be
> distressed (Rabow and Lee 2012). The diagnosis of
> advanced or metastatic disease, itself, is distressing,
> but when the cancer is no longer treatable, an existen-
> tial crisis is not uncommon.

They somehow managed to get up the rest of the stairs, stopping every now and then for Trudy to catch her breath. Eli was panting by the time they reached the top and he needed to hold onto the wall as they moved slowly to their bedroom. He got to the bed and lay down immediately, too tired to even get out of his clothes. He lay on top of the covers and Trudy covered him with a blanket. She barely managed to get into her pajamas before she too lay down and was asleep in seconds.

The next morning, Trudy woke with a start. There was a sound com-ing from the en-suite bathroom that scared her. As she stood up, she saw that Eli was not in bed, which meant that the sound was coming from him and something bad had happened. The bathroom light was off, and it took a few seconds for her eyes to adjust. Eli was lying on the floor, curled up and cradling his head in his arms. There was blood on the shower door and the front of his T-shirt was wet. The unmistak-able smell of urine reached her nose and she covered her mouth with her hands to stop herself from screaming. She reached for a towel and knelt to help Eli, who was sobbing, his shoulders shaking.

Despite her medical training, Trudy did not know what to do first. She tried to ask Eli what had happened and where it hurt, but he did not respond. As she knelt over him, she saw that he had hit his head on something. The wound on his head was no longer bleeding and he would have a horrible bruise there soon, but that was the least of it. He had wet himself but it was not clear to her if that happened before or after he fell.

"Eli, listen to me . . . please let me help you get up. You can't stay like this."

He didn't acknowledge her, but he started to sit up. He was still crying, but at least now he had stopped sobbing out loud. Trudy braced herself against the bathroom wall and helped him stand up, his legs were shaking, but at least he was upright. They shuffled to the bed where she helped him take off his wet T-shirt. He managed to get himself under the covers where he lay on his back, his eyes closed and his breathing heavy.

Trudy wanted him to go to the hospital for a CT scan, but Eli refused. He couldn't remember exactly what had happened, but he was embarrassed about wetting himself and just wanted to be left alone. Trudy was not going to let that happen and, for the rest of the day, she kept a close eye on him. She cleaned the bathroom while he slept, and when he woke after an hour, she insisted that she was going to help him shower. Eli grumbled about this but he was comforted that she would be close by; he would not admit that to her, of course!

To her relief, Eli seemed none the worse for wear; no bones were broken and he did not seem to be concussed. He stayed in bed most of the day, but he was able to read his book and he ate half a sandwich for lunch. She was nervous about him coming down the stairs in the late afternoon, but he insisted and she hovered behind him as he very slowly negotiated his way down. It was obvious that the effort was exhausting, and he sank into the couch in the den with a sigh.

He refused dinner, and so Trudy ate alone at the kitchen table, each mouthful of soup requiring effort to swallow. She was worried about Eli, and whether she was going to be able to cope with him at home for much longer. Her back still ached from the day before and helping him off the bathroom floor that morning had certainly not helped.

It is challenging to take care of someone whose health is deteriorating. Most family caregivers are not trained to provide the kind of care that the man may need. Depending on where you live, resources and support may not be easily available.

Over the next weeks, Eli grew weaker; he spent most of the day in bed, and Trudy was exhausted. John came by a couple of times a week, but he did not provide much help. He spent thirty minutes with his father but grew frustrated because Eli was too tired to talk and often fell asleep mid-sentence. Trudy had been giving Eli his pain medication on a regular basis; she wanted him to be as pain-free as possible. But that came at a cost; he slept a lot and wasn't eating much at all.

Erin rarely came to visit. John made excuses for her, but the truth was that she was so upset about Eli's condition that she would rather not see him so sick. John stopped by to see his father before or after work, and because Erin kept away, her in-laws hardly saw Samantha. This hurt Trudy deeply. She tried talking to John about this and all he said was that she should talk to Erin. Trudy was reluctant to do this; her relationship with her daughter-in-law was tenuous and she didn't want to make things worse. Eli asked almost every day when he was going to see Samantha, who was now two years old. John had brought her to visit one Sunday and seeing the little girl and hearing her talk made Eli smile for what seemed like the first time in months. But the following weekend, John came by alone, and when Trudy asked him where Samantha was, John told her that his wife believed that seeing Eli had upset the child. Trudy was flabbergasted and angry at the same time. If Erin loved Eli so much, then why would she deny him the joy of seeing his only grandchild? She didn't have the energy for a fight with Erin, or John for that matter, so she backed off.

The days stretched into weeks, and Trudy grew even more exhausted. She was barely sleeping and she felt on edge all the time. She was shocked when someone from Dr. Stone's office called to ask why Eli had missed his appointment the previous day. Trudy did not recall that he had an appointment; the last time they saw the oncologist had been the month before when he had increased Eli's pain medication and called in a new prescription. She was embarrassed that she had missed the notification about the appointment and as she thought about this, she realized that she had forgotten a lot lately. She had not paid the credit card the month before and the interest charges were astronomical! She was too tired to think about what else she might have missed.

When you are overwhelmed with responsibilities when caring for a spouse who is ill, tasks that you would usually do without even thinking can be forgotten. When you add lack of or poor sleep to the challenges of caregiving, functioning on all levels, mental and physical, will be affected.

She explained to the young woman from Dr. Stone's office that Eli was very weak and that she was not sure she would be able to get him out of bed, down the stairs, and into the car, but she knew that Eli needed medical attention.

"Oh, it sounds like your husband is not doing well," the woman replied.

Trudy kept quiet. She knew she needed help to take him to see Dr. Stone, but what was she supposed to do?

"Let me get you the number for a private medical transportation company. A lot of our patients use this service. They are reliable and they will take good care of your husband."

At last, someone was going to help! Within minutes she had the phone number of the transportation company and an appointment with Dr. Stone the next day. She wasted no time in making arrangements to get Eli to the doctor's office. Now she just had to explain this to Eli, and she was worried he was going to make a fuss.

When she entered their bedroom, Eli was sleeping. He slept most of the time now, and he barely moved when Trudy touched his arm. His eyes fluttered open and he tried to smile, but his lips were cracked. Trudy immediately felt guilty; she had not bothered to put something soothing on his lips. She was out of her depth doing this caregiving, and it was work. As a pediatrician, she had never had to do anything like this, and she felt helpless. She whispered to Eli that she had made arrangements for him to go to see Dr. Stone. She was expecting him to object, but he just patted her hand where it lay on his arm.

The next morning, the transportation she had arranged for arrived at the exact time she had requested. The two men who knocked on the door were polite and looked professional. They asked her if they would need a wheelchair or a gurney, but Trudy did not know the answer. She had managed to get Eli dressed; it was a struggle to get him into sweat-pants and a T-shirt, but she had done it. The men greeted Eli and asked him if he could walk. He seemed confused and looked over at Trudy expectantly, as if she would know the answer to their question. The men assessed the situation quickly; one of them went out to their vehicle and returned with a small wheelchair. They lifted Eli carefully without much effort, placed him gently in the wheelchair, and then carried him down the stairs. Trudy followed behind, her eyes following their every move. They were efficient and careful, and she said a silent "thank you" to the young woman who had suggested this.

They didn't have to wait more than a few minutes before they were ushered into an examination room at Dr. Stone's office. A nurse who introduced herself as Jodi asked them some questions; Eli had dozed off and Trudy tried her best to answer. She felt uncomfortable talking for Eli, but he seemed unaware of where he was. The nurse thanked her and said that Dr. Stone would be with them soon.

Dr. Stone entered the room within minutes. He talked to Eli, who answered him very briefly; he was not in pain, but he was very tired. He refused to be examined so the physician turned to Trudy and asked her what she thought.

"He sleeps most of the time. I give him the pain meds as prescribed and he seems to be comfortable. I'm not sure what else I'm supposed to do . . ." She was about to start crying so she stopped talking.

"How are *you* doing?" Dr. Stone asked quietly.

Trudy could only shrug her shoulders. She didn't want to let him see how upset she was. She was a highly trained medical professional who was not coping! This was so embarrassing.

Dr. Stone had seen this before, a family caregiver who was feeling hopeless and overwhelmed. It didn't matter that Trudy had medical training, she was now someone whose spouse was nearing the end of his life, and she needed help. "Do you think it's time that you got some help?"

Trudy nodded. She felt relieved that someone had asked the question. She was not coping, that was clear to the oncologist, and as he said the words, she realized that it was accurate. She really wasn't coping, as much as she tried to hide it.

"I'm going to make a referral to our palliative care team, and you can decide with them what you want to do. Your husband may choose to be admitted to the hospital at some time in the future, or you can keep him at home with support. It's up to you but I think this is the right way to go."

Trudy agreed to the referral and, as she nodded, felt as if a weight was lifted off her shoulders. She had thought this for some weeks, but admitting it, even to herself, felt like she was giving up. And perhaps she was, but she could not go on like this. She was tired, more tired than she could remember, and she knew that things were going to get more challenging in the days ahead.

The focus of palliative care is on management of pain and other symptoms that are causing distress. Being referred to palliative care services does not mean that death is imminent; some people receive this care so that they have the best quality of life possible.

Dr. Stone renewed Eli's prescription for pain medication and Jodi, the nurse who they had seen earlier, gave Trudy her contact information in case she had any questions. She told Trudy that a nurse from the palliative care program would call within twenty-four hours to set things up.

The transportation team was waiting for them when they left the office. Trudy felt better than she had in months; she now had a plan and a way forward. The drive home went quickly, and the two men carried Eli up the stairs and helped him into bed. Trudy offered them a tip, but they refused. She had tears in her eyes as she walked them to the door. It was their job but to her it felt like a gift.

Eli was fast asleep when she entered their bedroom; the trip had been exhausting for him. Trudy lay down next to him and fell deep asleep. She was woken by the sound of her cell phone ringing downstairs. By the time she found her phone, the call had gone to voice mail. The message was from one of the palliative care nurses; her name was Maggie and she wanted to arrange a time when she could visit them to plan for Eli's care. Trudy called back immediately and Maggie agreed to come to the house the next morning. Trudy felt so much better; the nap had done her a world of good and she was looking forward to meeting the nurse and getting some help.

Trudy called John to tell him what was happening. He didn't have much to say about their visit to the oncologist but promised to bring Samantha with him when he came to visit on the weekend.

The next morning, Maggie, the nurse, rang the doorbell five minutes before the arranged time. She started to apologize but Erin interrupted her.

"No need to apologize, I've been waiting for you!"

Trudy ushered Maggie into the living room. They sat down and Maggie started to explain what she did and how she might help the couple. She appeared to be in her forties, and when she smiled, her eyes wrinkled at the corners. Her voice was friendly, even though she asked very direct questions. After they had talked for almost forty-five minutes, she asked Trudy if she could meet Eli.

"He sleeps most of the time," she replied, "But of course, let's go upstairs."

When Trudy introduced Maggie to Eli, he managed to open his eyes and reached out a hand to shake hers. His hand was shaking, the tendons and bones stretching the skin. Maggie took his hand and covered it with her other hand. She gave it a gentle squeeze and told him that she was there to help him and Trudy. Eli nodded his head, almost as if giving permission to both Maggie and his wife, and then he was asleep again.

Maggie and Trudy went back downstairs. They didn't speak until they were once again seated.

"It must be a lot, going up and down those stairs all the time." Maggie's voice was gentle.

Trudy nodded. It *was* hard, and her back ached all the time now. She was helping Eli in and out of bed to use the bathroom, and having to go up and down the stairs to their bedroom wasn't helping. She had to check on him every hour during the day, and there were times when she stood at the bottom of the stairs, not sure that she was going to be able to climb them again. She confessed this to Maggie, and much more. She had not had a decent night's sleep in months, and she was not sure how much more she could handle.

"The first thing I would like to do is get a hospital bed brought in. That will help with transferring your husband in and out of bed. Is there a bathroom on this floor? Okay, good. And we can get a plastic urinal for him as well. That will lighten your load, too, if he can use that sometimes. Would that be okay?"

Trudy was embarrassed that she had not thought of this herself. After all, she was a doctor!

Maggie seemed to read her mind. "When you are the caregiver, you may not think of these things. That's why I'm here! To relieve you of some of the decision-making, especially about the small things . . ."

Maggie was making notes as they talked and as she left, Trudy saw that she was talking on her phone, making calls to arrange for what they had discussed. She had assured the nurse that, for now, she wanted to try and manage things herself but she promised that she would ask for more help if it got too much.

> While many partners feel that they have to cope and that they have to be able to care for their partner 100 percent of the time, this is often not possible. With some rest and respite from doing it all, all the time, you may find yourself spending more quality time with your partner.

To Trudy's surprise, Erin was with John and their daughter when they came to visit that weekend. John and Erin went to say hello to Eli while Trudy played with her granddaughter. Shortly after they went upstairs, the doorbell rang and there was Maggie, coming to check on Eli. Trudy had not expected a visit on the weekend and was unsure how to act; she had not told her son that she and Eli were now receiving help, and she did not know how he was going to react.

She did not have to wait long to find out; John came downstairs and she introduced him to Maggie. His response was to grunt and then he turned around and went back upstairs. Trudy started to apologize for his rudeness but Maggie quickly changed the subject. She had lots to tell Trudy; the hospital bed was going to be delivered early on Monday morning and she had also ordered a wheelchair, just in case Eli was able to go outdoors. She told Trudy that she would not interrupt Eli's visit with his son and daughter-in-law but would be back the next day.

As soon as Trudy closed the door behind Maggie, she heard footsteps coming down the stairs. Samantha was sitting in her highchair where Trudy had put her while she was talking to Maggie. The little girl was contentedly pushing the remains of a cookie around the tray and greeted her parents with a loud "hi!'" Neither of them seemed to notice; they both started to talk very loudly to Trudy.

"Who is that person and why was she here?" John's voice was loud enough to startle his daughter.

"Why did you let a stranger into the house instead of asking me to help?" Erin's voice was angry and accusing.

Trudy was speechless. Why were they so angry at her? It was not that they had offered any help; Erin had not visited for weeks, and John's visits were brief. They did not seem at all concerned about Trudy's well-being and this is what hurt the most. It had not been easy for her to accept help, but knowing that Maggie was there had given her renewed energy to look after Eli. Instead of responding to them, Trudy pointed at Samantha, who was looking at them, her eyes filling with tears and her mouth open, just about to cry out loud. This stopped her parents in their tracks; Erin picked up the child and walked to the front door, John following close behind her. He turned around as he picked up his car keys.

"I don't know what to say, Mom . . ."

It is important for family members to understand what you, as the primary caregiver, are going through. You may think that they can see how tired you are or how difficult the situation is, but they may not see it.

The next morning, Maggie came back to the house. She wanted to be there when the hospital bed was delivered. She did not say anything about John's behavior, and Trudy was grateful for that; she did not know how she would explain his rudeness. The nurse asked if she could go up and talk to Eli; she suggested that Trudy have a shower in the guest bathroom while she was there and Trudy accepted the suggestion with relief.

Thirty minutes later, she felt like a new person; she had been having sponge baths because she was scared to leave Eli alone and out of earshot while she was in the shower. Maggie was sitting at the kitchen table, making notes on her iPad, her phone at her ear as she typed.

"Ah, Trudy, was the shower good?"

Trudy nodded.

"We need to talk . . . please sit. I made some coffee, if that's okay with you."

Trudy had not seen that she had done this and she poured herself a mug.

Maggie cleared her throat. "I talked to Eli for a little bit while you were in the shower. He didn't say much, but he was more awake than when I saw him the other day. Trudy, he knows that the end is near and he is worried that this is too much for you. He wants to go to hospice, he was clear about that, and he doesn't want you to be mad at him . . ."

Trudy immediately responded with a range of emotions. She was shocked that this is what he wanted but she was also immensely relieved. She felt guilty that he wanted this too; was she not providing him what he needed? She was sad that he knew that he was dying, although she knew that he must be aware of this. How could he not be? And she was scared that this was going to cause problems with John and Erin who did not seem to understand the situation.

Maggie seemed to know exactly what Trudy was thinking and feeling. "Would it help if I was there when you talked to your children?"

Trudy nodded. She needed a buffer for that conversation. A little later that morning, she called John and asked him and Erin to come over. Her son heard the tone in her voice and did not make an excuse. They came by just before dinner; they had asked Erin's sister to look after Samantha and so they were alone. They were surprised to see Maggie there, and Trudy did not give them an opportunity to say anything about the nurse's presence. Maggie had made some suggestions about how the conversation could begin, and Trudy followed those.

"John, Erin . . ." her voice was hesitant but she continued. "Your father has decided that he wants to go to hospice." She did not pause even though her son had opened his mouth to say something. "He knows that he is going to die soon and he doesn't want to do that here." She was crying as she said this, but she knew she had to finish. "I have been caring for him by myself until Maggie came, and I am exhausted and I just can't do this anymore. This is the best decision for your father and I, and if you can't accept it . . ." Trudy could not continue; her shoulders were shaking as she sobbed.

"Hospice? What is that?" John's voice was loud. Erin was talking at the same time.

"What do you mean he's dying? We thought, we hoped, that this was just a bump in the road. We didn't realize that this was the end!"

Trudy had stopped crying and she looked at Erin in disbelief. How could she think that? She had been to visit shortly before, and Eli had slept through most of the visit. Did she not notice how thin he was? How could think that he would get better?

Maggie interrupted them and explained about hospice. Her voice was even and this seemed to calm everyone down.

Hospice refers to programs that support individuals to plan for the end of life, respecting their wishes and providing support to the family. Hospice care can be provided at the person's home or at a hospice center. Specialized care by professionals, usually nurses and aides, is available 24/7.

John and Erin had started to cry. Trudy sat silently, her eyes on the tabletop. She felt guilty that she had not been more open with her son and daughter-in-law about Eli's condition, but how could they not have seen? She was grateful to Maggie for supporting her; she was not sure she could have done this without her help.

"Please ask me any questions you have." Maggie spoke softly as she passed tissues to the couple. They did not have many questions; they seemed to be in shock. All their anger and confusion melted into sadness as the realization set in that Eli did not have much time at all. The couple stood up and readied themselves to leave; they had not left Samantha with anyone before and they were worried that she was upset. John hugged his mother for a long time before they left. The hug was an apology, an offer of support, and an expression of love.

CONCLUSION

Not everyone will survive their cancer, and disease progression can occur over many months or years. Prostate cancer is often described as the "good" cancer because most men do not die from it. Anyone who has had cancer, or who has a loved one with the disease, knows that no cancer is "good." Families may be at odds when it comes to the end-of-life wishes of their loved one. Honest sharing of feelings and clarification of what the man with cancer and his primary caregiver need with family members is very important.

Reflective Questions

After reading this chapter:

- What could have been done to avoid the shock that Eli's son and daughter-in-law experienced when they learned that their father was going to die?
- When is a good time to involve support like palliative care?
- How could Trudy have prevented almost burning out while caring for her husband?

REFERENCES

Rabow, M. W., and M. X. Lee. 2012. "Palliative care in castrate-resistant prostate cancer." *Urologic Clinics of North America* 39 (4): 491–503. doi: 10.1016/j.ucl.2012.07.006.

Chapter Thirteen

Self-Care

"It's You I'm Worried About"

The partners of men with prostate cancer may deny themselves the support and opportunities for self-care in their attempt to support the man. This is not a good idea—as they tell you on airplanes, you need to put on your own oxygen mask before helping others! In this final chapter, the story of one man's partner highlights what can happen when they put their own needs behind that of the man with prostate cancer. Their emotional and physical health suffers and their ability to be supportive decreases. Eventually, the partner agrees to seek help and discovers a range of activities that are helpful for their own self-care.

Lorne and Bev Brandford have been married for ten years; this is a second marriage for her. Bev's late husband died of brain cancer at the age of thirty. They had three young daughters at the time, and Bev raised them on her own until she met Lorne. He had never married, and he quickly fell in love with both Bev and her daughters. The girls are now young women with lives of their own; the twins are thirty years old and both are teachers. The youngest is twenty-five and a speech and language pathologist. They live close by and spend time with Lorne and Bev on the weekends.

Lorne and Bev met at the high school where he is a math and science teacher; Bev is the administrative assistant to the principal at the same school. Lorne says that he fell in love with her the moment he first saw her. It took her a little bit longer to notice Lorne and to agree to a date; she thought that she would be alone forever. Her girls were teenagers at the time, and Bev's focus was on them. It was not easy being a single parent, especially with three teenage girls, but she was used to being on her own. A romantic relationship was not on her radar at all, and initially she was confused by Lorne's attention. Her daughters encouraged her to go on a date with him, something that she regarded as a little strange. But they had few memories of their father, and they wanted her to be happy. So she went on a date with him, and then another, and soon they were spending a lot of time together. He got on well with her girls, and they with him. They got married a year after they started dating; Lorne wanted a "proper" wedding, even though she preferred something small and private. The girls were her bridesmaids and Lorne looked so happy that day that she let go of her misgivings about the wedding and enjoyed herself.

Lorne was diagnosed with prostate cancer six months ago. It was not a good time to have surgery, if ever there is a good time, but in the middle of the COVID-19 pandemic, it could not have been worse. Bev was not allowed to visit him in the hospital, and she barely slept while he was there. He came home on the second day after the surgery and Bev almost wept when she saw him walking through the doors of the hospital toward the car. He decided to have surgery because that meant less time in the hospital than if he had a course of radiation. He also wanted his treatment over and done with during the summer when schools were closed. He had been teaching remotely for the whole of the last semester of the school year, and he wanted nothing more than to be back in the classroom in the fall. Bev, on the other hand, was hoping that they would not go back to in-person classes. She liked working at home, and that way she could keep an eye on her husband.

She couldn't help thinking about her first husband and how each time he was discharged from the hospital, he was a little bit weaker, and their time together a little shorter. The grief she felt during his illness and after his death had dulled over the years, but Loren's diagnosis pulled her back into the fears and distress that she thought she had put behind her. Her experience with her late husband as he went through his cancer treatments had made her vigilant for any signs that something was wrong. She had watched him like a hawk, but it changed nothing. His cancer grew and his symptoms worsened. And then he died. She was going to make sure that this was not going to happen again.

Past experiences are not predictive of the future, especially when it comes to cancer. Every cancer is different and everyone's response to the cancer and its treatment is different too. That includes the experience of spouses. It is common for partners of men with cancer to be vigilant for any signs of change in the man's condition.

The first few weeks that Lorne was home after his surgery were good. The COVID-19 pandemic meant that they weren't going out much, so Lorne spent a lot of time reading, something that he didn't have much time for during the school year. Bev had time to cook healthy meals and lost a few pounds, something that pleased her. The girls visited on the weekends, as they usually did; they loved him and were happy to just hang out. She worried about him, and even though he told her he was fine, she monitored him constantly. She watched him as he slept, looking for any facial expression suggesting he was in pain. She wouldn't allow him to do anything around the house, not even making himself a sandwich for lunch. This irritated him and he told her so; she didn't want them to have a fight, so she backed down. But soon she went back to preparing him his meals before he could try to do anything for himself. He eventually gave up and let her do everything for him. Bev was exhausted, both physically and emotionally, but she would not stop. He could see how tired she was, but when he asked her if she was okay, she wouldn't tell him the truth; all she said was, "I'm okay, it's you I'm worried about."

Soon it was the start of the new semester and Bev and Lorne returned to work. Bev was worried about this because COVID-19 was rampant in the state where they lived. Mask wearing was encouraged in the school where they worked, but not many of the students were wearing them and those who did often had their nose exposed. The teachers complained that they had to raise their voice to be heard through the mask, and so many gave up wearing them. Bev was concerned that Lorne was doing this too, but when she asked him, he got irritated.

Then Lorne got sick. He woke in a pool of sweat in the middle of the night. Bev woke up too, his shivering had disturbed her, and she fumbled around in the bathroom, trying to find a thermometer. She eventually found it, but by that time, Lorne was out of bed, pulling the bedsheets off the mattress. He would not allow her to take his temperature, but she could see that he had a fever; his face was flushed, and he was still shivering. She rushed to get clean sheets out of the linen closet and they changed the bed linen in silence. His damp T-shirt and shorts were lying on the floor where he had undressed. He had replaced them with the first thing he had found in his drawer, and Bev almost laughed when she saw what he was wearing. He had found an old sweatshirt that had a rip under the armhole, and he was wearing swimming trunks! Bev did not say a word as she gestured for him to get under the covers. She took his temperature and her eyes widened when she saw the reading; it was 101.4°F, so he definitely had a fever!

"You need to take something to get your fever down. I'm going to get you some medication . . ."

Lorne nodded his head. He was lying with the covers up to his chin and was still shivering. Bev almost ran to the kitchen where they have a supply of pain killers and other assorted medications. Her hands shook as she opened the bottle of Tylenol; he usually had a glass of water on his nightstand but she couldn't remember if it was empty, so she grabbed a bottle of water out of the fridge. Lorne refused to take the pills with the ice-cold water and the glass on his bedside table was empty. So back to the kitchen she went, where she took another bottle of water from the stock in the pantry. When she got back to the bedroom, she could not find the pills! She had the bottle in the pocket of her housecoat and she poured out two more pills and watched as Lorne swallowed them.

Now she was too wide awake to sleep, so she went back to the kitchen and filled the kettle to make herself a cup of chamomile tea. Her mind was racing; did he have COVID-19? She stood at the kitchen counter and took a couple of deep breaths. He needed to have a test, but where did they have to go to get one? This was not something she just knew; so far, they had managed to keep mostly to themselves and so she had not paid much attention to testing locations. She tried to calm herself and think rationally; where was she most likely to find the information she needed? She glanced at the clock on the wall; it was 3 a.m. so she could not call any of her daughters. Then she remembered something about a website that had information about COVID-19 testing. She quickly logged on to the computer and found the information; there was a drive-through testing site about five miles away and it opened at 6:30 a.m.

She checked on Lorne every thirty minutes through the rest of the night. Once the pills kicked in, his fever had dropped and he was sleeping peacefully. Bev knew that she was not going to be able to get back to sleep, so she sat in the living room, the TV on with the sound turned down. Shortly before 6 a.m., she woke her husband.

"Lorne, sweetheart, we have to get you tested for COVID-19. I guess I need to test too. There's a testing place not far from here, and we need to get going. Please get up!"

Lorne shook his head and burrowed deeper under the sheet, but Bev was insistent. They were both due at school before 7:45 a.m., but now she would have to call the principal and tell her what was going on. The last thing she needed was to have to fight with Lorne! She left the bathroom door open as she brushed her teeth. There was no time for a shower now, so she wet her hair to make herself somewhat presentable. She banged the closet doors and slammed drawers as she dressed, trying to get him up. Eventually, Lorne got out of bed and got dressed; he kept on the ratty sweatshirt and pulled on a pair of jeans from the laundry basket. He didn't do anything else and Bev could smell his foul breath; at least the mask would deal with that! She said nothing as she handed him a clean mask and they left the house.

The process of testing for COVID-19 was mercifully quick and within twelve hours they got the results; they were both infected. For the next two weeks they hunkered down; Lorne's fever had dropped, and he had lost his sense of smell and taste. He used the time away from school to continue reading, and he was happy to be able to do that. He didn't complain about anything related to his surgery, so she assumed that he was okay. Bev, on the other hand, was not well. She had lots of aches and pains and was exhausted. She slept fitfully at night, and she was often awake for long periods. When she couldn't sleep, she watched old movies on her iPad and worried that this would wake Lorne, so she left him in their king-size bed. The mattress in the guest bedroom was old and her back ached even when she was lying down. She worried constantly about Lorne and whether COVID-19 was a risk to his recovery from the surgery.

Being diagnosed and treated for cancer is a life-altering event for both the man and his spouse. When this is complicated by another illness, the burden increases exponentially. The COVID-19 pandemic has increased uncertainty and added additional burdens and responsibilities on caregivers.

Bev did not ask her daughters for help; she was worried that they could become infected if they had any contact with her or Lorne. She ordered groceries online and had them delivered to the house. She tried to cook every day despite having no appetite, and she felt guilty about the amount of food she was throwing away. Lorne was still having regular night sweats and the amount of laundry she did every day was overwhelming. She usually enjoyed this task—she found folding the warm clothes, sheets, and towels comforting—but now it felt like too much and there was so much more to wash, dry, and fold.

Two weeks later, they went back to work; they had both recovered from COVID-19 according to the information they had been given when they went for testing. Lorne seemed to be handling things better than she was. He had breaks between classes, but she had to be at her desk all the time. The phone rang constantly, and students came in seemingly every few minutes to ask questions or to report that they did not feel well. She was still not sleeping properly, and her exhaustion made her irritable and incapable of showing patience to anyone. It came to a head at the end of her first week back when the school principal asked her to organize a virtual meeting for later that day.

"You want me to *what*?" Bev's voice was so loud that one of the teachers walking past the office stopped to see what was happening. "It's almost lunchtime, and I haven't had time to go to the restroom." Bev had tears running down her face, but she did not notice.

Ms. Bridges ("Shelly" to the staff), the principal, was looking at Bev with a horrified expression on her face. "Bev, in my office, please!"

As she followed the principal into her office, Bev felt her face turning red and hot. She was embarrassed and confused; where did her response come from? She had never spoken so rudely to anyone at the school, least of all Shelly, who was a fair and decent boss. The principal sat down on one of the chairs facing her desk and motioned for Bev to sit next to her. Bev could hardly make eye contact with her; she sat down slowly, her eyes on her lap.

"What's going on, Bev?" the woman asked quietly, "This is not like you."

Bev struggled to keep her voice steady. "I am *so* sorry, Shelly! My response was out of line, completely and totally. Can you forgive me?"

"It's not a question of forgiveness, Bev," the principal continued. "Something is wrong, and I want to help . . ."

Bev had started crying again; her voice was halting as she spoke. She was not sure that she wanted to share how she was feeling with the school principal. "Maybe it's COVID-19 . . ."

She knew that this was an excuse, but she didn't know what else to say. She had notified the school that both she and Lorne had tested positive for COVID-19 and then she had called again to say that they were coming back to work when the required period of isolation had passed. They wanted to retire in the next few years and needed to save as much as they could while they were both working.

"Maybe it is, but I think there's something more," replied the principal. "I've had some complaints from parents about your communication with them. One of the parents also complained about the way you spoke to their child. Yes, I know that the parents often complain about things without merit, but what bothers me is that this is so out of character for you."

Bev was staring at the principal as she spoke. Parents had complained about her? That was awful.

"And you've let some of your other work slide too, Bev. The minutes from my meeting with the Student Council were late, and there were a lot of errors in there. This is not like you."

Bev was horrified; she prided herself on her work, and to hear that she had given her boss inferior work was profoundly embarrassing.

"I would like you to see someone, to talk to someone. I've asked the school guidance counselor for some names of people she would recommend." The principal's voice was gentle, and Bev knew in her heart that Shelly was trying to help.

"Okay, I'll do that. Thank you."

Accepting the need for support or professional help is not always easy, particularly for those who are used to being capable and able to cope. Adjusting to new and uncertain circumstances is not easy, even for those who are usually in control of everything!

The principal wanted Bev to go home after their talk, but Bev needed to wait for the end of the school day to ride home with Lorne. She returned to her desk and tried to focus on catching up on the work that she had missed when she was off sick. It was hard to concentrate; Shelly's words were still in her head and she felt so ashamed. It was all she could do to stop herself from crying. Thankfully, only three students came to the office, and she was able to answer their questions quickly. The phones were also quiet for a change, and there were just two hours until the end of day. She was quiet in the car going home, and Lorne didn't seem to notice that she was out of sorts.

Over dinner that evening, she told Lorne about her conversation with Shelly. She was surprised at his response; he was not outraged and told her that he agreed that she should see a counselor.

"That's not a bad idea."

"But . . . I'm so embarrassed . . . and we can't afford counseling."

"Of course, we can! We could afford my surgery and that cost thousands! You've been dealing with so much! First me, and then COVID-19, and don't think I don't know that you haven't been sleeping!"

How did he know about her sleep, or rather lack of sleep? She was still sleeping in the spare bedroom and she thought he didn't know that she spent most of the night watching movies.

"How did you know?"

Lorne stood up, moved toward her, and pulled her out of the chair. He put his arms around her and held her tight. She could feel his heart beating and she relaxed into his hug. She immediately felt guilty that he was taking care of her when she should be taking care of him. He was the one who had surgery for cancer and she hadn't once asked him how he was feeling since they went back to work! She started to apologize, but he "shushed" her and continued to hold her close. It felt so good to be held by him, and as he continued to hug her, she closed her eyes and, for the first time in what felt like ages, she took a deep breath.

The next morning before school started, she called the number of the counselor that Shelly had given her. She left a message and got a call back mid-morning. The counselor introduced herself as Andrea and suggested a couple of appointment times that were available the next week. Bev agreed to see her the following Tuesday afternoon. She knew that if she thought about it or checked with Lorne about taking the car, she would chicken out. She quickly emailed Shelly that she would need to leave early that day and she got an immediate response with a smiley emoji instead of words.

Her daughters came over for a visit the following weekend. It was lovely to see them after the almost three weeks that they had kept away because of Bev and Lorne having COVID-19. Sunday was a beautiful fall day, and Bev and the girls went for a walk around the neighborhood. Many of the houses were decorated for Halloween and they reminisced about the years where they had to make do with just an orange porch light instead of decorations because, after their father died, there was no money for extras. By the time Bev married Lorne, the girls were teenagers and didn't care about decorations.

They walked three across, with Bev in between the twins and Rosie, the youngest, lagging a bit behind. She was looking at something on her phone and almost bumped into the other three, who had stopped walking.

"Mom . . . I—I mean we—Adele and I, want to say something." Anna's voice was hesitant.

The twins were named Adele and Anna and Anna was the most outspoken of the three siblings. She was the younger of the twins by thirty minutes, and although she had always been smaller than her older twin, she was also the bravest.

Bev held her breath; what was Anna going to say?

Adele interrupted her sister as she often did. "Mom, we've noticed that you're not the same. You're quieter and you haven't called any of us like you usually do.. Are you okay? Are you sick? I thought that your COVID-19 was over."

Bev looked at each of her daughters and she thought how she could answer the questions. She did not want to burden them with her problems; they all had their own challenges while working during the pandemic. But she knew that they would worry even more if she didn't tell them the truth. "It's nothing serious, girls. I'm fine . . . okay, that's a slight exaggeration! I've not been sleeping well and I guess COVID-19 took more of a toll on me that I thought. I was worried about Lorne and his surgery and then we got COVID-19 and well . . . I'm exhausted and I guess I'm not coping well."

"Oh, Mom, why didn't you tell us? We could have helped." Rosie and Adele spoke at the same time.

"It's okay . . . really, I'm going to see someone on Tuesday." Bev could barely get the words out but she needed to reassure them. For the years that she was alone with them, she had always told them that things were fine, that she was okay, that they would always be okay. She never wanted them to think that something could happen to her and so she had put on a brave face even when things were definitely not okay.

Her reassurance seemed to help them; the girls put their arms around her and each other as they stood in the middle of the street. For a minute, Bev flashed back to the days when their arms reached around her waist, but now they were taller than she was. It felt good to have their arms around her, and she leaned into the hug for as long as they stood still. They walked home with lighter spirits; Rosie and Anna had a fallen leaf fight and Adele looked on in disgust; she was the more serious one and she often took on the teacher role with her siblings.

On Monday, Bev tried to concentrate on her work, but her mind kept going to the appointment the next day. She worried about it even though she knew that going was for her own good. She had never needed this kind of help and knowing that she needed help was distressing. She thought about cancelling but resisted the impulse. She didn't want the principal, or Lorne, to get mad at her, and her daughters seemed so relieved when she told them about the appointment.

It is not unusual to feel scared or embarrassed that you need help from a professional. Counselling with a professional involves identifying what *you* need to address, whatever is bothering you.

Bev's heart was beating fast as she climbed the stairs to the second floor of an old rowhouse where the counselor had her office. She was a little short of breath when she knocked on the door, following the instructions that were posted there. As she lowered herself onto a chair that was placed beside the door, it opened and a woman stood there, a smile on her face.

"You must be Ms. Brandford. I'm Andrea, please come in!"

The office was small with a desk in one corner; a couch and one other chair took up most of the space. There was a box of tissues on the couch and one small cactus plant on the corner of the desk. Bev sat down on the edge of the couch; she was uncomfortable at the prospect of baring her soul to this stranger.

"Let me explain who I am, my experience with clients, and how I practice before we start . . ." Andrea quickly explained that she was a social worker with ten years of experience working with clients of all kinds. She particularly liked working with women, and her focus was on helping her clients help themselves. She smiled as she spoke and her warmth put Bev at ease. Soon Bev was telling her everything, even some things that she had not realized were bothering her. Bev spoke for twenty minutes without interruption; the words poured out of her and she didn't notice that she was crying off and on. She hadn't noticed taking tissues, one by one out of the box, and then balling the wet ones in her lap.

"It sounds like you've been through a lot."

Bev sighed. Yes, she had been through a lot, and it was only in the recitation of the last months that she acknowledged the worry and fatigue that had affected her every waking moment. She had been worried about Lorne from the moment he received the cancer diagnosis and, of course, when he had the surgery. She had not been able to visit him while he was in the hospital, and this only increased her anxiety. Despite his assurances that he was doing okay, Bev worried about his recovery. He gave no signs that anything was wrong but still she worried. And then they both got COVID-19 despite doing everything right, or at least that is what she thought. And going back to school was scary; many of the teachers and the students were not vaccinated and maybe they could get sick again! There was so much about this pandemic that she wasn't sure about.

"Have you heard the term 'emotional labor'?" asked the counselor.

"No, what is that and what does it have to do with me?"

"The common understanding of emotional labor is the unpaid and usually invisible work that we do to keep things stable in the home. It's about how we work hard to keep everyone around us happy, safe, and comfortable."

"So, what's so bad about that?" Bev's response was defensive; wasn't that what women are supposed to do?

"I'm not suggesting that you have been doing anything wrong," Andrea ignored the tone in Bev's words. "It's just that we, and by 'we' I mean mostly women, take on a whole lot of emotions and that has consequences. Your worry about your husband is not wrong, but one of the consequences is that you are not sleeping well. And despite the fact that you also had COVID-19 and may still be experiencing symptoms, you continue to care for others, your boss and the students and their parents, putting your own needs in second place."

Bev sighed. That made sense but what was she supposed to do about it? Before she could ask the question, Andrea answered her.

"Self-care is so important when you are taking care of others. There are several things that you can do to help yourself when you are helping someone else. Are you open to hearing about them?"

Bev nodded; she appreciated that Andrea did not tell her what to do.

"The first thing is that *you* need to get enough sleep. I know that is not easy, but lack of sleep impacts our ability to cope and to do many of things we need to do in order to take care of ourselves!"

Bev gave a small smile; she knew she was not sleeping well, but what was she supposed to do? Worrying about not sleeping was not going to help!

"Something else that can help is not going full tilt and trying to do everything. You need to pace yourself so that you conserve energy for the important things. Do you have friends or family members that can help you with the daily tasks that use energy and that can be done by someone else? Like laundry, for instance. We often decline offers of help because we want to show everyone that we are coping."

Bev gave a short laugh. That is exactly what she did! The girls had offered to cook some meals for them after Lorne came home from the hospital, but she had refused.

"You know how good it feels to help someone else?" Andrea was looking at Bev, and Bev found herself hanging on every word. She nodded, yes it did feel good.

"Well, why not give someone else the pleasure of helping *you*?"

Now Bev felt embarrassed. She had declined all offers of help and she was not sure why she had resisted those offers. Did she think that she was the only one who could wash the dishes or do laundry? It would have been so helpful if she had only asked the girls for some help when she was looking after Lorne in those days when he was just back from the hospital.

"What are some of the things you enjoy?" asked Andrea.

"I really enjoy going for walks, mostly by myself. I put on my earphones and listen to music or podcasts and before I know it, I've been gone for almost an hour. I haven't been able to do that for such a long time. First, I was looking after Lorne and then I got COVID-19, and I just don't have the energy!"

"Please don't blame yourself for not being able to keep this up!" Andrea's voice was kind. "Getting some physical activity every day helps with so much, but it's often the first thing that falls by the wayside when we are overwhelmed. And it's the one thing that really helps to reduce fatigue!"

"It also helps me to cope at school," Bev added. "The phones never stop, and the kids are constantly interrupting me. I know that is why I have a job—to respond to the kids and the parents—but often I don't get a minute's peace!"

"That must be difficult, Bev," commiserated Andrea. "You have a high-stress job with many demands. And you seem to be a bit of a perfectionist." Andrea smiled at Bev as she said this. Most of her female clients had similar stories and it was often hard to get them to understand that taking care of themselves enables them to take care of others. The old adage about putting on your own oxygen mask before helping others is true in caregiving. If you are not taking care of yourself, you will not be able to help your spouse/partner.

Caring for someone during the COVID-19 pandemic has increased stress for many. Women and racial or ethnic minorities are especially impacted, and there are physical, emotional, financial, and social outcomes of caring for a loved one during the COVID-19 pandemic.

The two women continued to talk for the rest of the appointment. Bev found it easy to open up to the social worker. She was not at all judgmental and she really listened to what Bev was saying. She made suggestions, but they did not feel like orders. She even seemed to understand Bev's reluctance to take a break from work.

"The work we do is an important part of our identity, I understand that. But you have two jobs, like many of us! And on top of that, you have been sick too. You can't continue to do everything without some help. So, what are you willing to do to help lighten your load?"

Bev thought about this for a while. She could not give Andrea an immediate answer and as she started to tell the social worker this, Andrea looked at the clock on the wall.

"Oh dear, our time is up. I'm so sorry but perhaps this will give you some time to consider what your next steps are going to be. Would you like to meet with me again? Maybe in a week or two?"

"Next week would be great. This has been really helpful!"

Bev walked back to her car; she felt the beginnings of a sense of hope for the first time in months. She felt that Andrea had truly understood her and most of what she had said made sense. As she drove home, she thought about what she needed to do to lighten her load and the first thought was never saying "I'm okay, it's *you* I'm worried about," again.

CONCLUSION

Caregiving for someone who is sick can be a full-time commitment. It is often done out of love and concern but also with the attitude that you are the only one who can do the care taking. This may end in harm to your physical or mental health and may have consequences for your work and other relationships. Asking for help may not be easy, but being asked for help can feel really good. Denying those who love and support you the ability to help you is not a good thing. Asking for help when you need it is a form of self-care.

Reflective Questions

After reading this chapter:

- How easy or difficult is it for you to ask for help?
- How did the COVID-19 pandemic affected your daily life?

- What lessons have you learned from living through the pandemic?
- What routine tasks could you assign to someone else while caring for your partner?
- What strategies have you tried to improve or increase your self-care practice?

Index

About the Author

Anne Katz, PhD, RN, FAAN, works as a clinical nurse specialist and certified sexuality counselor at the Manitoba Prostate Centre in Winnipeg, Canada. She supports men with prostate cancer and their partners through prostate cancer, from diagnosis and into survivorship. This book is her fifteenth publication and a complete revision of the first edition of *Prostate Cancer and The Man You Love* (2012).

CPSIA information can be obtained
at www.ICGtesting.com
Printed in the USA
BVHW041215310722
643205BV00010B/3